anatomy of
FUNCTIONAL
TRAINING

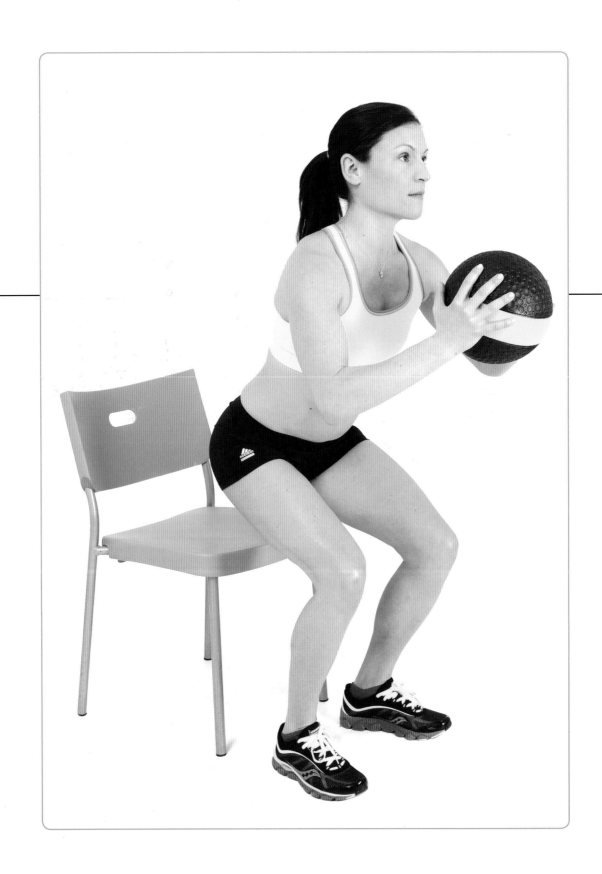

anatomy of
FUNCTIONAL TRAINING

Katerina Spilio &
Erica Gordon-Mallin

BLOOMSBURY

LONDON · NEW DELHI · NEW YORK · SYDNEY

Note
While every effort has been made to ensure that the content of this book is as technically accurate and as sound as possible, neither the authors nor the publishers can accept responsibility for any injury or loss sustained as a result of the use of this material.

Published by Bloomsbury Publishing Plc
50 Bedford Square
London WC1B 3DP
www.bloomsbury.com
First edition 2013
Copyright © 2013 Moseley Road Inc.

ISBN 978-1-4081-8998-6

Moseley Road Inc.
President: Sean Moore
General Manager: Karen Prince
Art Director: Tina Vaughan
Production Director: Adam Moore

Editor: Erica Gordon-Mallin
Designer: Heather McCarry

Photographer: FineArtsPhotoGroup.com
Models: Joseph Benedict, Jillian Langenau

This book is produced using paper that is made from wood grown in managed, sustainable forests. It is natural, renewable and recyclable. The logging and manufacturing processes conform to the environmental regulations of the country of origin. Printed and bound in China by Oceanic Graphic Printing (OGP)

10 9 8 7 6 5 4 3 2 1

CONTENTS

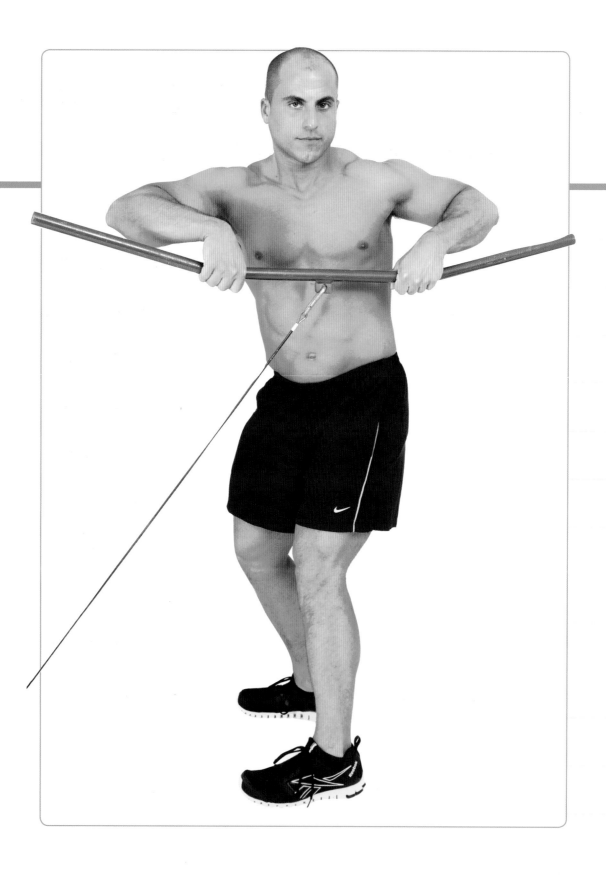

INTRODUCTION: TRAINING FOR LIFE

Functional training is for anyone inspired to get into shape from head to toe. It is for those who want to throw a ball harder, develop a smoother tennis stroke, or swim more laps – in the fast lane. It's also for people of any age or fitness level who want to feel good walking up stairs, running for the bus, or reaching for the top shelf … and cultivate a beautiful body along the way.

In functional training, muscles matter. The technique recognises that the myriad muscles in our bodies work together; when one fires, other parts of the body react. Functional exercises use numerous muscle groups along multiple planes of motion. The moves reflect real-life situations, incorporating lateral and horizontal movement to hone balance, flexibility and stamina.

FORM AND FUNCTION

In functional training, quality trumps quantity. Your goal is not to rush through as many repetitions as you possibly can in a knee-jerk way. Instead, it is to do as many repetitions as you can while maintaining optimal form.

If you notice your form starting to deteriorate – your shoulders creeping up toward your ears, for instance, or your torso twisting to one side – you should switch to a different exercise rather than adding more repetitions of the same exercise. Aim for a range of different exercises so that many muscle groups are engaged.

BUT WHY?

Why is form so important? Isn't calorie burn the same, regardless of how we move?

If you are sedentary, just getting off the couch and moving around – regardless of what you do or how you do it – will improve your fitness levels, and you should congratulate yourself for it. But when fitness is an important part of your life, whether this is due to athletic pursuits or persistent pain, it makes sense to do it right. This is true for various reasons.

For one, good form is kinder to your spine. When you pay attention to your form, keeping the muscles in your legs, arms, and core engaged as you perform most of the exercises in this book will help to protect your body from the back pain that can accompany sudden bursts of exercise, not to mention the countless other movements like bending, listing and twisting that

daily life demands.

Working a range of muscles at the same time helps to counteract muscular imbalance; a common condition in which one muscle becomes overdeveloped and compensates for other muscles, which then weaken – sometimes spurring discomfort and pain. For instance, if you attend spinning classes often and exclusively, you may find your quadriceps getting stronger while your hamstrings only get a secondary challenge. This could lead to knee pain or problems. A remedy might entail adding an exercise like Dead Lift to your routine in order to balance the new strength in your quads.

On top of all this, the functional training technique of working multiple muscles as you focus on flexibility, balance and range of motion gets you a better body. The multitasking approach helps you to tone up and get in shape more effectively, justifying those hours in the weight room or on the fitness mat.

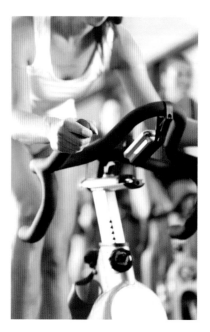

Counteract muscular imbalance by adding complementary exercises to your routine.

TIPS FOR BETTER FORM

To give your form a boost, tune in to these tips – which apply to most exercises in this book.

- Avoid clenching or collapsing parts of your body. When performing ArmReach Plank, for instance, try adding a very subtle bend in your elbows so that your muscles, not your ligaments, do the work. And avoid locking your joints, whether they are joints you are moving or static ones. Your goal is dynamic engagement, rather than getting comfortable in a position and resting there.

- Pay attention to how you come out of each repetition. All too often, we lift weights above our heads and then let them fall down carelessly, jerking our spines and wasting a chance to strengthen arms and abs in the process. But coming out of an exercise is an opportunity to engage muscles, and paying attention to it maximises benefits and avoids injury.

- Aim for balance. For every abduction, your body will benefit from an adduction, and for every flexion, an extension. In this way you will develop muscles equally and to their full potential.

- If an exercise causes stress or strain, take a week or two off from performing it. Then, ease into it again at an easier level and see how your body reacts before increasing, for instance, the amount of added weight or the number of repetitions.

- In most exercises and in everyday life, picture your navel being pulled inward toward your spine. Your belly shouldn't bulge outward, but take care not to 'suck in' either at the expense of proper breathing.

- Knee soreness is never desirable. Try placing a rolled up blanket beneath your knee(s) when kneeling or squatting if contact with the floor feels uncomfortable. Never use a foam roller on your knee; instead, roll above or below the knee area.

- Naturally, the muscles in your spine form an S-shaped curve. This is sometimes referred to as the neutral curve of your spine. Optimal posture involves supporting this neutral curve. When possible, therefore, your back should be neither hunched forward nor arched.

- Study how you sit, whether at the office or driving: do you lean to one side, stressing your abdomen or straining your lower back? You may need to add some lumbar support. If you find yourself twisting to one side, make a conscious effort to correct this imbalance through exercise. In addition to cultivating a sense of centeredness, this will help to prevent strain and possibly injury down the line.

- As a general rule, inhale to prepare, and then exhale as you carry out an action such as lifting or reaching. Soon you'll get a rhythm going, and will find that your breath helps you through your workout. Breathing while you move releases tension and affords you optimal control of your body. Deep inhalation and full exhalation exercises the lungs, increasing their capacity. Breathing, in short, benefits your functionality. Let your belly rise as you inhale and flatten as you exhale.

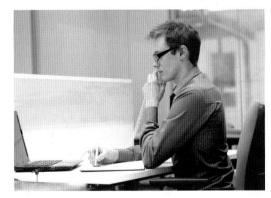

Study how you perform everyday tasks to see which functional training exercises can benefit you.

A FUNCTIONAL LIFESTYLE

Our bodies weren't designed to sit around. As mammals, our bodies evolved to climb trees and mountains, forage and hunt for food, and fight for physical survival every day. Ironically, though, the lack of exercise in our contemporary daily routines has many fighting for survival again, combatting problems like type II diabetes and high cholesterol.

Through exercising regularly, especially in an aware, functional way, we are in effect returning to what's natural. To see big benefits, aim for three 45-minute exercise sessions per week. Then, over time, try for even more: the results can be transformative, leading to lower cholesterol and body fat as well as better mood.

Although the step-by-step instructions in the following pages tell you to perform a certain number of repetitions, this is only a guideline and should not be the focus of your training. Instead, aim to carry out all of your repetitions with optimal form. Once you feel your back arching, your abs bulging outward, or your arms flailing around, you may not be getting the most from the workout regardless of how quickly you move or how many reps you complete.

MEASURING PROGRESS
If you're not racing through your Functional Burpees or banging out a bunch of Seated Russian Twists, then how do you measure your functional training progress?

Over time, you should see an increase in the number of repetitions that you can carry out with proper form. For a person of average weight, performing 30 repetitions of an exercise like Mountain Climber exhausts muscles. Doing more and more reps with good form leads to muscle conditioning and greater endurance. Taking a shorter break between exercises brings your heart and your lungs into the work, helping you reap the cardiovascular

benefits as well.

With form at the forefront of your mind, you can use the number of repetitions, and sometimes even speed, as a way to gauge your progress. As you practise functional training, try asking yourself: is this becoming habit? Is my muscle memory getting ingrained with good habits, so that I feel a centeredness, flexibility, powerfulness and even grace as I move through the daily tasks I used to ignore?

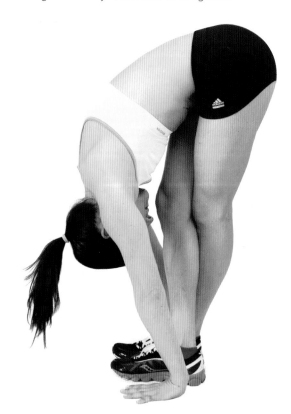

Try stretching a little more deeply each time you perform Iliotibial Band Stretch.

EQUIPMENT

Various pieces of equipment can augment your functional training. In the following pages, for instance, you'll encounter the following.

medicine ball – a weighted ball used to strengthen and condition by adding weight to traditional exercises.

Swiss ball – an inflatable ball used to engage pelvic and abdominal muscles as well as provide instability in exercise routines

foam roller – a cylinder approximately 3 feet long by 6 inches wide used for releasing muscles

body bar – a weighted bar, used for resistance training, stretching and balancing

step – a sturdy jump platform used for dynamic and plyometric exercise

dumbbell and barbell – bars with weighted discs or balls at either end, used for muscle conditioning; a barbell is larger and heavier

resistance band – a supple band that is often held taut and pulled against to enhance muscle-toning benefits of exercise

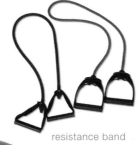

resistance band

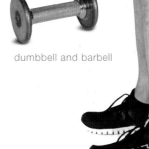

dumbbell and barbell

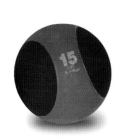

medicine ball

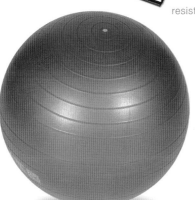

Swiss ball

body bar

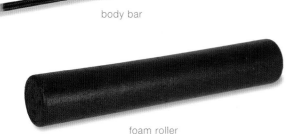

foam roller

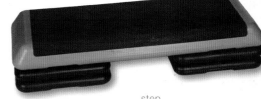

step

Catch yourself engaging your core muscles, maintaining a neutral S-curve in your spine, or bending at the knees to pick up a box, and you'll know your regimen is working. Aim for flexibility and a fuller range of motion; your palms may not rest flat on the ground during Ilitoibial Band Stretch at first, but with practice you will reach further and further, until suddenly there you are.

Some of the exercises contain elements that may look familiar. However, it is worth taking time to revisit them. You may be tempted to rush through a set of Push-up Walkouts, for instance – but tuning into the functionality of your muscles will help you rediscover the movement.

It's worthwhile to watch yourself working out. Trying looking into a mirror at first, or ask a friend about your form. Make sure your toes stay on the floor, your neck doesn't arch uncomfortably, and your belly stays pressed toward your navel with your abs engaged as you move. Think about the muscles in your arms, your legs, your core, and even your glutes staying engaged and working together – and you will likely feel the benefits of Push-up Walkout in a new way.

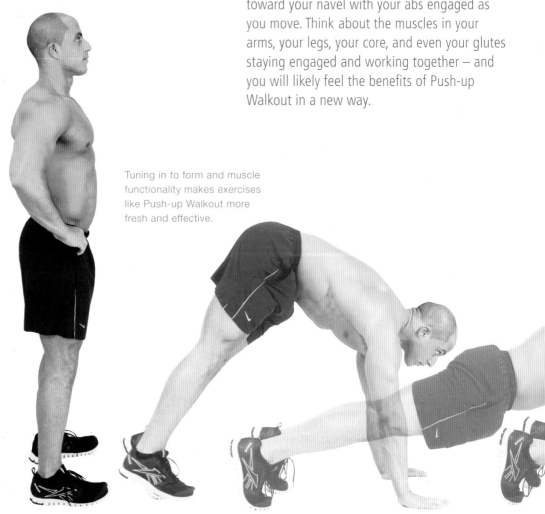

Tuning in to form and muscle functionality makes exercises like Push-up Walkout more fresh and effective.

FUNCTIONAL FUELING

Diet is an important complement to your exercise regimen. As with your fitness efforts, think of diet in terms of functionality. Beyond its myriad pleasurable qualities – very important in themselves! – food is there to fuel your lifestyle.

There is no one-size-fits-all way to eat healthfully, as all bodies have individual needs. It is important to get regular blood tests to identify cholesterol levels and determine whether you are getting enough of various vitamins. Also, try tuning in to your body's sensitivities: if you find

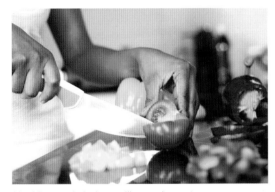

Healthy meal choices will complement your functional training regimen.

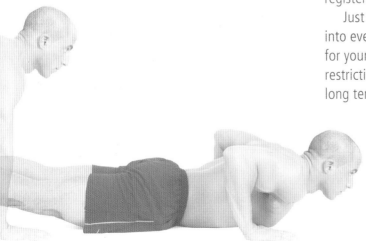

yourself getting sleepy after lunch every day, the blood sugar spikes caused by the carbohydrates in your sandwich or the processed sugar in your dessert may be to blame. Experiment with dietary changes, bearing in mind that how you feel is very important.

WEIGHTY ISSUES

For many of us, getting leaner is a top priority. A 1-pound weight loss involves a calorie deficit of 3,500. Shedding weight lies in burning more calories than we ingest. Alongside your exercise program, try keeping a food journal. You may find that the simple act of recording your food intake exerts a big effect on how much you eat.

One tip: when a craving strikes, don't deprive yourself or 'eat around' the craving. Instead, indulge – starting with a small portion. You know that feeling halfway through a big, indulgent meal when it stops being fun and you start to feel weighed down? Try pausing at that point. So often we lose track of our satiety levels; it actually takes our bodies 20 minutes to digest a meal and to fully register what we've eaten.

Just as functional training should be woven into everything you do, your diet should work for your entire lifestyle and should not be so restrictive that it can't be sustained over the long term.

TREAT YOURSELF WELL

Listening to your body and responding to its needs is an important part of functional training. Follow these tips to help your body function for you. Bonus: you'll combat exercise fatigue.

• Warm up. Run in place, dance, walk briskly around the garden or down the street, set up an obstacle course in the kitchen – wwhatever gets your muscles warm will do the job. Aim for a minimum of 5 minutes, though 15 minutes is ideal.

• Keep breathing as you exercise. You'd be surprised how easy it is to hold your breath while working hard – in fact, it's natural to do so when performing a new or stressful task. And your breath can become shallow for numerous reasons; a sedentary lifestyle, anxiety, and nasal congestion can all play a role. If you catch yourself holding your breath or breathing shallowly, remind yourself to breathe fully, naturally, and with a sense of ease.

• If injury occurs, use functional training techniques to help with healing. For instance, problems with the iliotibial (IT) band, part of the tensor fascia latae, can cause lateral knee, hip or back pain so if you have pain there make sure to include that stretch. In addition, many of these exercises and stretches can be incorporated into a physical therapy routine. Consult with your doctor or therapist to choose the proper exercises post-surgery or post-injury.

• Stay hydrated. If you start to feel thirsty, that means you are already approaching dehydration. Keep a water bottle within reach.

• After a workout, take time to cool down, stretch, and let your muscles release.

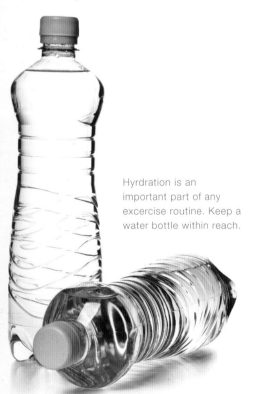

Hyrdration is an important part of any excercise routine. Keep a water bottle within reach.

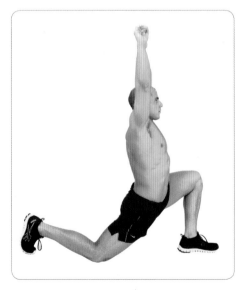

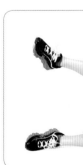

USING THIS BOOK

Consider this book your invitation to unlock the functionality of your whole body.

Start with Body-Weight Exercises, paying attention to the Do It Right and Avoid boxes. Once you feel comfortable with the form, move on to the Body-Weight Exercises to hone muscles, and to Resistance Exercises to tone up.

In the final chapter of this book, you will find Stretching & Releasing moves. Practise these on areas of the body that feel tight or painful under pressure; you may even feel some relief immediately after the exercise. Even releasing should carry a functional training twist. Think of your body as a unified whole rather than a collection of unrelated parts. For instance, during Tensor Fasciae Latae Roll, utilise the strength in your arms to modulate the amount of leg weight that is pushing into the roller.

In the following pages, you will find diagrams showing which muscles are called into play when you complete each exercise. As you work out, visualise your muscles not just 'firing' to power the movement but also staying engaged and dynamic as you work. In so many ways, these exercises carry intrinsic benefits as well as boosting your performance in sports, and the Benefits and Performance Boost sidebars illuminate these rewards.

At the very end of the book is a list of suggested workouts, which will help you boost posture, transition from a long day at work to a night out, and more. Above all, this guide to functional training is yours to explore. We wish you all the best.

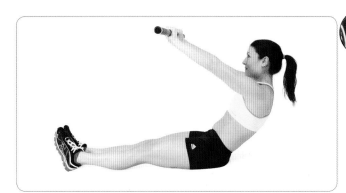

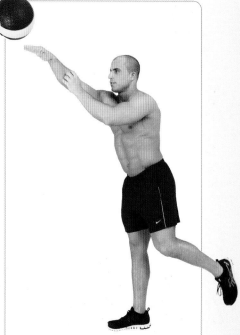

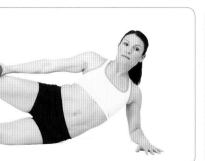

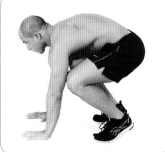

FULL-BODY ANATOMY

ANNOTATION KEY

* indicates deep muscles

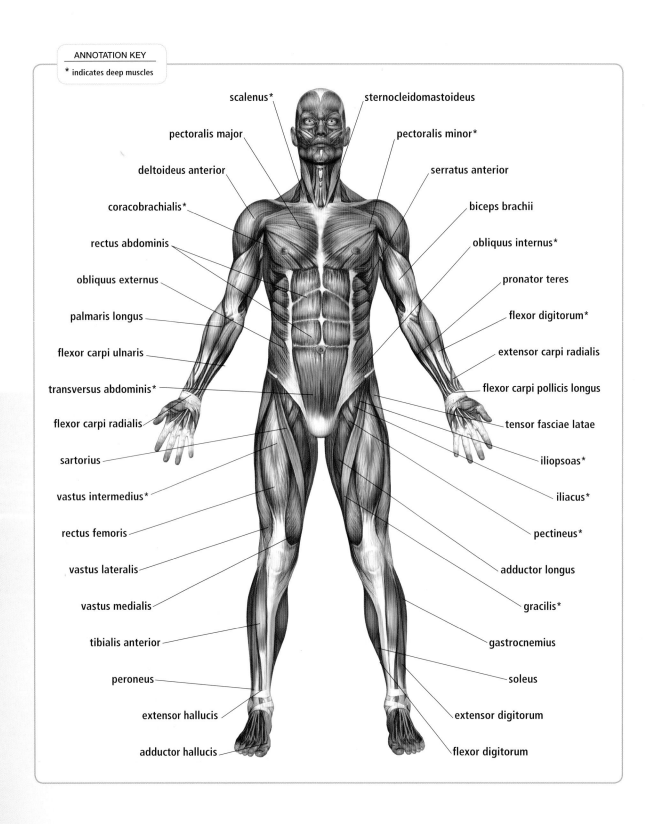

scalenus*

sternocleidomastoideus

pectoralis major

pectoralis minor*

deltoideus anterior

serratus anterior

coracobrachialis*

biceps brachii

rectus abdominis

obliquus internus*

obliquus externus

pronator teres

palmaris longus

flexor digitorum*

flexor carpi ulnaris

extensor carpi radialis

transversus abdominis*

flexor carpi pollicis longus

flexor carpi radialis

tensor fasciae latae

sartorius

iliopsoas*

vastus intermedius*

iliacus*

rectus femoris

pectineus*

vastus lateralis

adductor longus

vastus medialis

gracilis*

tibialis anterior

gastrocnemius

peroneus

soleus

extensor hallucis

extensor digitorum

adductor hallucis

flexor digitorum

semispinalis*

splenius*

trapezius

levator scapulae*

infraspinatus*

supraspinatus*

deltoideus medialis

teres major

deltoideus posterior

erector spinae*

subscapularis*

latissimus dorsi

teres minor

brachialis

rhomboideus*

brachioradialis

triceps brachii

extensor digitorum

anconeus

quadratus lumborum*

multifidus spinae*

gluteus minimus*

gemellus superior*

gluteus medius*

quadratus femoris*

piriformis*

obturator internus*

tractus iliotibialis

obturator externus

gluteus maximus

vastus lateralis

semitendinosus

gemellus inferior*

biceps femoris

adductor magnus

semimembranosus

plantaris

tibialis posterior*

gastrocnemius

flexor hallucis*

soleus

trochlea tali

flexor digitorum

adductor digiti minimi

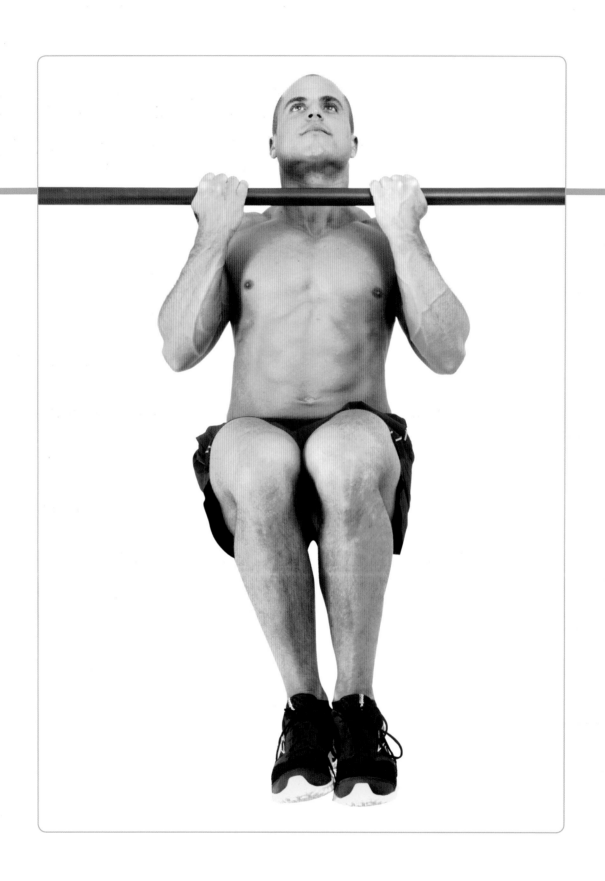

BODY-WEIGHT EXERCISES

Moving your body effectively is key to functional training. Explore the following exercises before you move on to add weight or perform resistance moves. In time, these exercises will help you to build endurance, flexibility, strength and stability – along with helping you to burn calories and tone. Remember to think of your body as a unified whole. Rather than isolating individual muscles as the rest of your body goes lax, you are aiming for total body engagement.

WARM-UP OBSTACLE COURSE

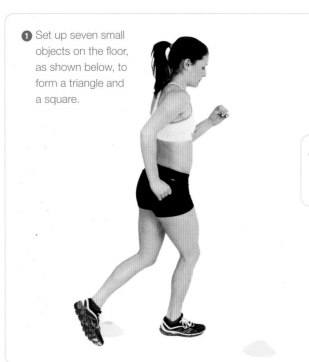

❶ Set up seven small objects on the floor, as shown below, to form a triangle and a square.

AVOID
- Stopping at any point.
- Moving too quickly throughout the course.

BENEFITS
- Warms up muscles
- Improves agility

PERFORMANCE BOOST
- Tennis
- All field sports

❷ Taking small, quick steps, step around all of the objects in the triangle.

❸ Stand in front of the square and jump forward to land in the middle of the square. Complete a jumping jack.

❹ Jump forward to land outside the square. Jog back to the beginning of the course and repeat.

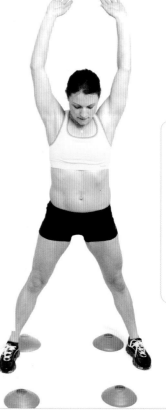

DO IT RIGHT
- Keep a steady pace as you move through the course.
- Take small steps, focusing on coordination.
- Stand upright.
- Keep your abdominal muscles pulled in and engaged.

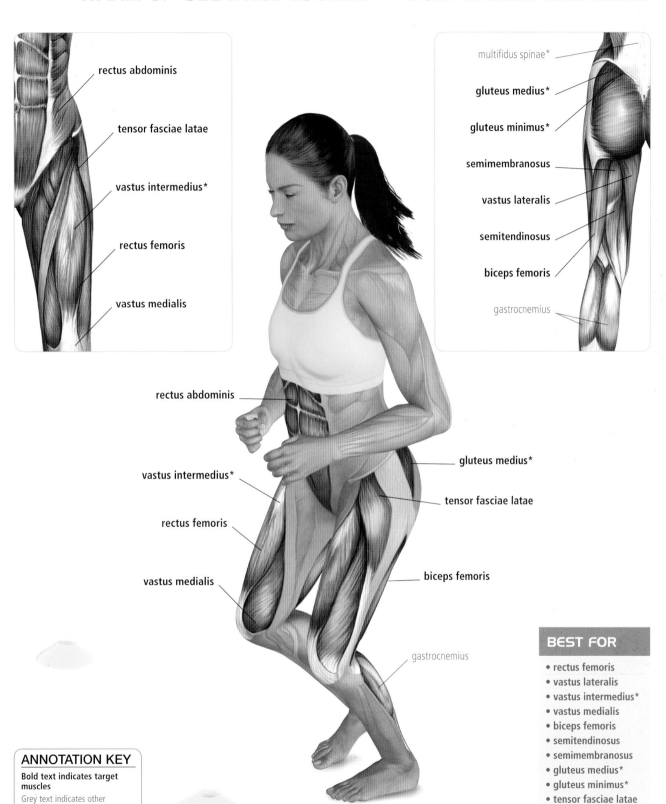

rectus abdominis

tensor fasciae latae

vastus intermedius*

rectus femoris

vastus medialis

multifidus spinae*

gluteus medius*

gluteus minimus*

semimembranosus

vastus lateralis

semitendinosus

biceps femoris

gastrocnemius

rectus abdominis

vastus intermedius*

rectus femoris

vastus medialis

gluteus medius*

tensor fasciae latae

biceps femoris

gastrocnemius

ANNOTATION KEY

Bold text indicates target muscles

Grey text indicates other working muscles

* indicates deep muscles

BEST FOR

- rectus femoris
- vastus lateralis
- vastus intermedius*
- vastus medialis
- biceps femoris
- semitendinosus
- semimembranosus
- gluteus medius*
- gluteus minimus*
- tensor fasciae latae
- rectus abdominis

DIAGONAL REACH

1. Stand with your feet hip-width apart and your arms at your sides.

2. Raise both arms upward and to the right to form a diagonal line. Follow your hands with your gaze. Return to starting position.

3. Repeat to the left side. Perform 12 repetitions.

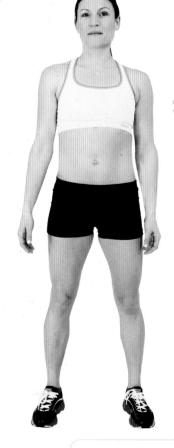

BENEFITS
- Stretches and strengthens the muscles used for twisting

PERFORMANCE BOOST
- Tennis
- Golf

AVOID
- Twisting your hips.
- Letting your abs bulge outward.
- Hunching your shoulders.
- Tensing your neck as you lift or lower your arms.

DO IT RIGHT
- Keep your abdominal muscles engaged.
- Keep your hips facing forward.
- Press your shoulders down.

BEST FOR

• rectus abdominis
• obliquus internus*
• obliquus externus

ANNOTATION KEY

Bold text indicates target muscles

Grey text indicates other working muscles

* indicates deep muscles

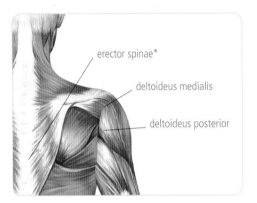

erector spinae*

deltoideus medialis

deltoideus posterior

MODIFICATION

Harder: Reach farther, bringing your arms to a steeper diagonal in one direction while raising the opposite foot off the floor.

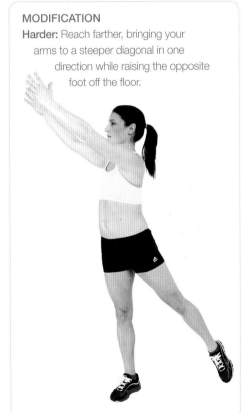

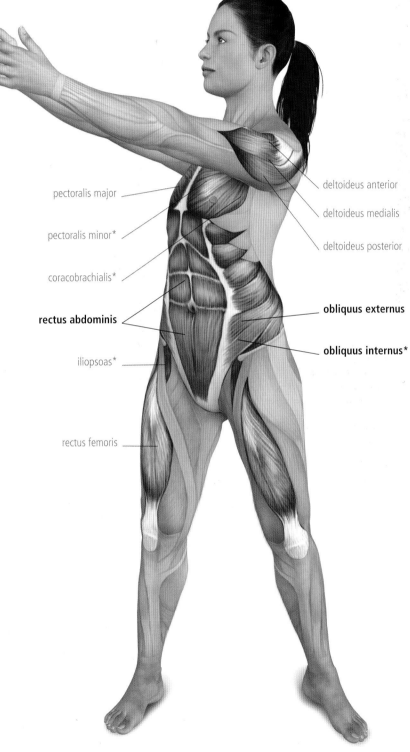

pectoralis major

pectoralis minor*

coracobrachialis*

rectus abdominis

iliopsoas*

rectus femoris

deltoideus anterior

deltoideus medialis

deltoideus posterior

obliquus externus

obliquus internus*

LATERAL-EXTENSION REVERSE LUNGE

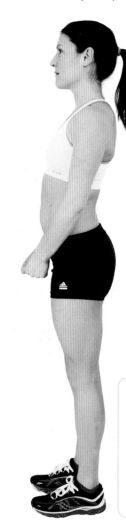

❶ Stand with your feet hip-width apart and your arms at your sides or on your hips.

❷ Step your right leg back, resting the top part of the foot on the floor.

❸ Bend both knees as you move into a lunge position. Lower your body, flexing your left knee and hip until your right leg is almost in contact with the floor. Raise your arms to the side until they are level with your shoulders.

❹ Return to starting position by extending the hip and knee of your left leg and bringing your right leg forward to meet your left.

❺ Repeat on the opposite side. Alternating, complete 10 on each side.

BENEFITS
• Strengthens gluteal and leg muscles

PERFORMANCE BOOST
• Baseball
• Rugby
• Soccer

DO IT RIGHT
• Keep your shoulders pressed downward.
• Keep your neck relaxed.
• Maintain upright form in your upper body as you lower and then raise your body.

AVOID
• Twisting either hip.
• Hunching your shoulders.
• Arching your back or hunching forward.

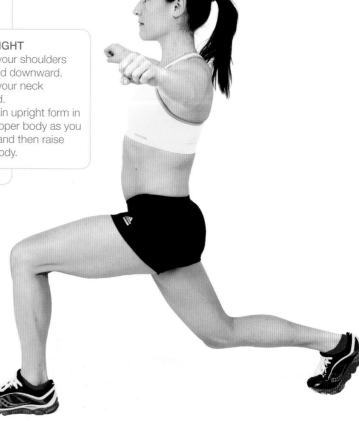

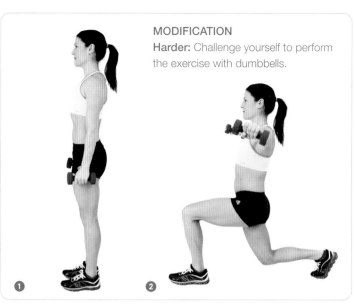

MODIFICATION

Harder: Challenge yourself to perform the exercise with dumbbells.

ANNOTATION KEY

Bold text indicates target muscles

Grey text indicates other working muscles

* indicates deep muscles

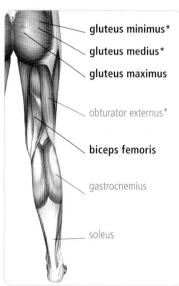

gluteus minimus*

gluteus medius*

gluteus maximus

obturator externus*

biceps femoris

gastrocnemius

soleus

BEST FOR

- rectus femoris
- vastus lateralis
- vastus intermedius*
- vastus medialis
- biceps femoris
- semitendinosus
- semimembranosus
- gluteus maximus
- gluteus medius*
- gluteus minimus*
- deltoideus medialis
- erector spinae*

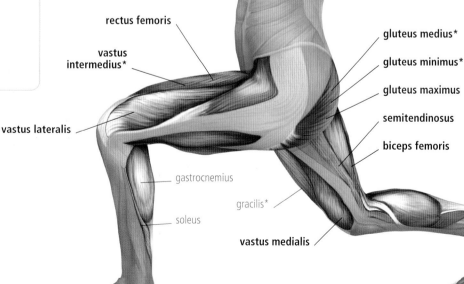

deltoideus medialis

erector spinae*

rectus femoris

vastus intermedius*

gluteus medius*

gluteus minimus*

gluteus maximus

semitendinosus

biceps femoris

vastus lateralis

gastrocnemius

gracilis*

soleus

vastus medialis

CHAIR PLIÉ

❶ Stand with your feet in a wide stance, with toes turned out and the chair in front of you.

AVOID
- Turning your toes out to the point where it is uncomfortable.
- Twisting to either side.
- Arching your back or hunching forward.
- Losing your balance by moving in a jerky manner.

DO IT RIGHT
- Keep your abdominal muscles pulled in.
- Keep your knees soft.
- Move gracefully and with control.

BENEFITS
- Engages and tones inner-thigh adductors
- Improves lateral movement

PERFORMANCE BOOST
- Tennis
- Football

❷ Keeping your knees aligned with your toes, bend your knees and lower your body into a squat position.

❸ Keeping your back straight, raise yourself back to starting position. Perform 10 repetitions.

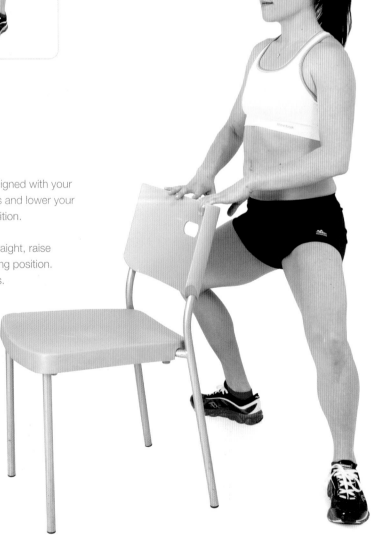

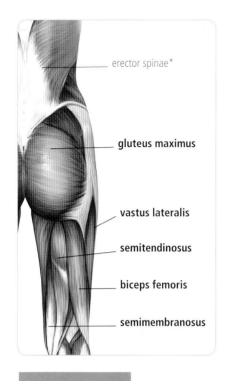

erector spinae*

gluteus maximus

vastus lateralis

semitendinosus

biceps femoris

semimembranosus

ANNOTATION KEY

Bold text indicates target muscles

Grey text indicates other working muscles

* indicates deep muscles

BEST FOR

- gluteus maximus
- rectus femoris
- vastus lateralis
- vastus intermedius*
- vastus medialis
- biceps femoris
- semitendinosus
- semimembranosus

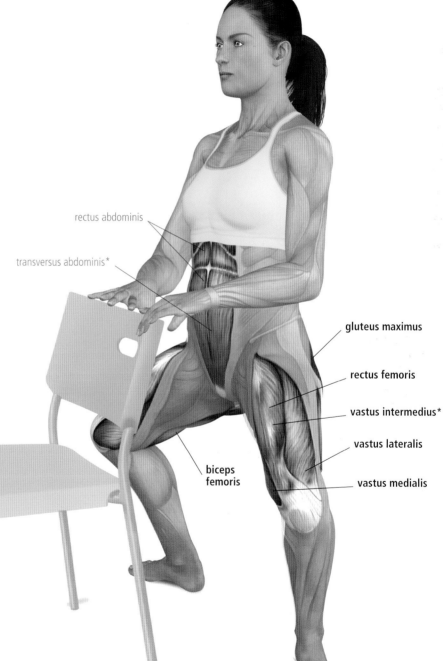

rectus abdominis

transversus abdominis*

gluteus maximus

rectus femoris

vastus intermedius*

vastus lateralis

biceps femoris

vastus medialis

CHAIR SQUAT

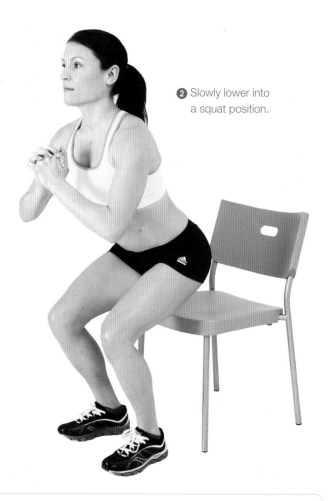

❶ Stand upright in front of the chair. Clasp your hands and position them in front of your chest.

❷ Slowly lower into a squat position.

BENEFITS
• Restores mobility after injury
• Counteracts sedentary lifestyle

PERFORMANCE BOOST
• Tennis
• Basketball
• Field sports

❸ Continue lowering until you are resting on the chair.

❹ With control, rise back up to the starting position and repeat, aiming for 10 repetitions.

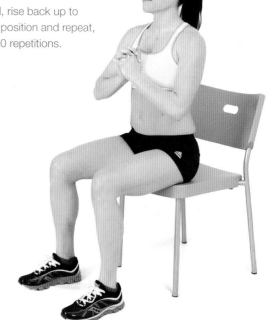

AVOID
• Arching your back or hunching forward.
• Tensing your neck.
• Hunching your shoulders.

DO IT RIGHT
• Gaze forward.
• Keep your back straight.
• Engage your abs.

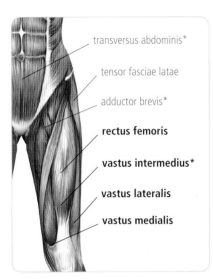

- transversus abdominis*
- tensor fasciae latae
- adductor brevis*
- **rectus femoris**
- **vastus intermedius***
- **vastus lateralis**
- **vastus medialis**

BEST FOR

- rectus femoris
- vastus lateralis
- vastus intermedius*
- vastus medialis
- biceps femoris
- semitendinosus
- semimembranosus
- gluteus maximus

MODIFICATION

Harder: Challenge yourself by holding a medicine ball throughout the exercise.

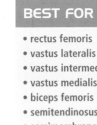

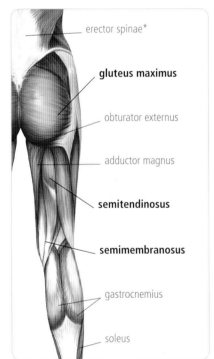

- erector spinae*
- **gluteus maximus**
- obturator externus
- adductor magnus
- **semitendinosus**
- **semimembranosus**
- gastrocnemius
- soleus

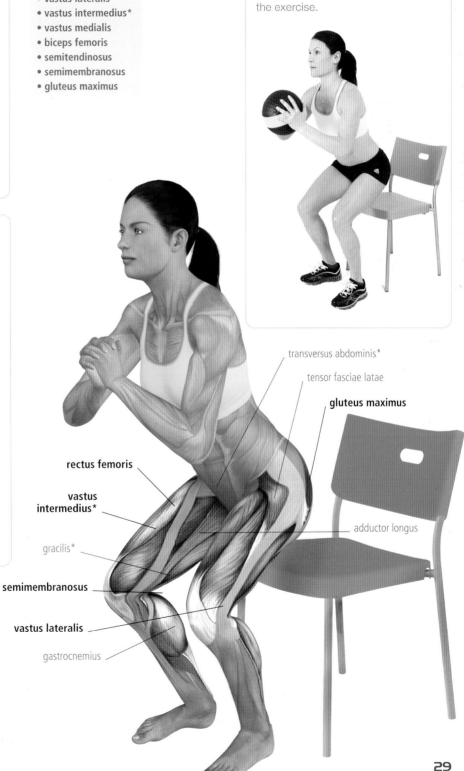

- transversus abdominis*
- tensor fasciae latae
- **gluteus maximus**
- adductor longus
- **rectus femoris**
- **vastus intermedius***
- gracilis*
- semimembranosus
- **vastus lateralis**
- gastrocnemius

ANNOTATION KEY

Bold text indicates target muscles

Grey text indicates other working muscles

* indicates deep muscles

SPLIT SQUAT WITH OVERHEAD PRESS

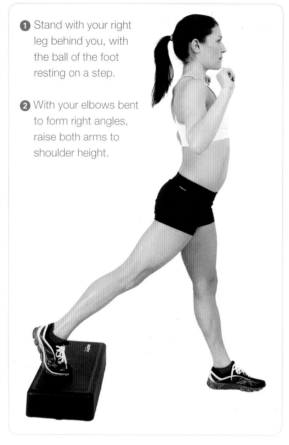

1 Stand with your right leg behind you, with the ball of the foot resting on a step.

2 With your elbows bent to form right angles, raise both arms to shoulder height.

3 Bend both knees into a split squat position. Simultaneously, extend your arms over your head.

4 Return to starting position, and then repeat. Aim for 10 repetitions. Then, switch sides and perform 10 more repetitions with the other leg behind. If desired, repeat the whole sequence 2 more times.

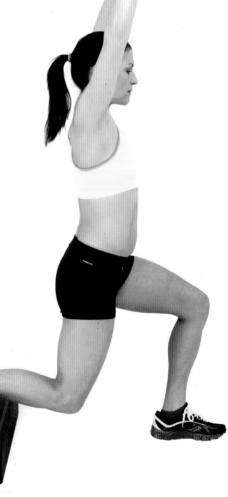

BENEFITS
- Strengthens glutes, quadriceps, hamstrings and trapezius
- Improves range of motion throughout body

PERFORMANCE BOOST
- Basketball
- Field hockey
- Rugby

AVOID
- Arching your back as you raise your arms.
- Letting your abs bulge outward.
- Tensing your neck.

DO IT RIGHT
- Keep your back straight and your core upright.
- Press your shoulders back and down.

MODIFICATION

Harder: Hold dumbbells throughout the exercise.

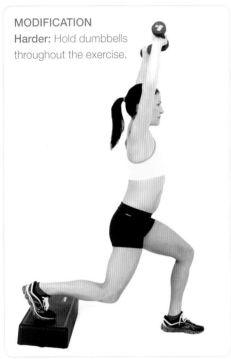

ANNOTATION KEY

Bold text indicates target muscles

Grey text indicates other working muscles

* indicates deep muscles

BEST FOR

- rectus femoris
- vastus lateralis
- vastus intermedius*
- vastus medialis
- biceps femoris
- semitendinosus
- semimembranosus
- gluteus maximus
- gluteus medius*
- gluteus minimus*
- deltoideus anterior
- deltoideus medialis
- deltoideus posterior

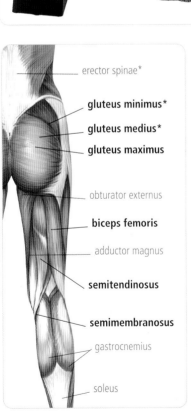

erector spinae*

gluteus minimus*

gluteus medius*

gluteus maximus

obturator externus

biceps femoris

adductor magnus

semitendinosus

semimembranosus

gastrocnemius

soleus

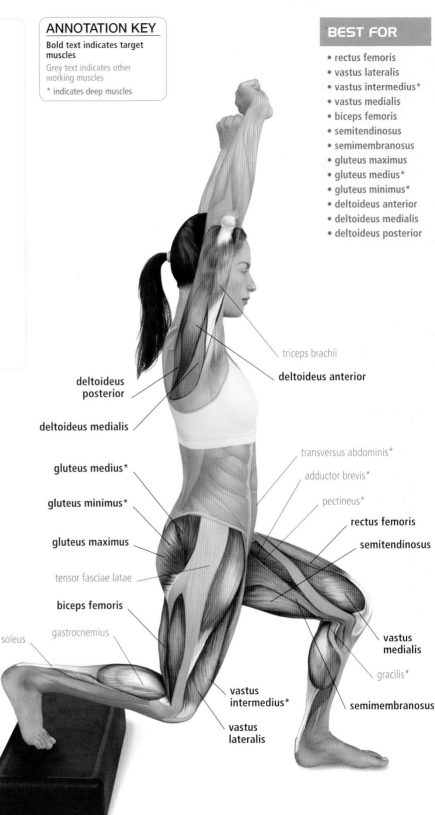

triceps brachii

deltoideus anterior

deltoideus posterior

deltoideus medialis

transversus abdominis*

adductor brevis*

pectineus*

gluteus medius*

gluteus minimus*

rectus femoris

semitendinosus

gluteus maximus

tensor fasciae latae

vastus medialis

biceps femoris

soleus

gastrocnemius

gracilis*

semimembranosus

vastus intermedius*

vastus lateralis

FUNCTIONAL BURPEE

❶ Stand with your feet hip-width apart and your arms above your head.

DO IT RIGHT
- Challenge yourself by maintaining a quick pace.
- Contract your abdominal muscles in the plank position.

AVOID
- Moving through the positions so quickly that you compromise your form.

BENEFITS
- Warms up muscles
- Improves coordination
- Strengthens and tones abdominal, chest and leg muscles
- Plyometrically integrates explosive movement with cardiovascular exercise

PERFORMANCE BOOST
- All field sports

❷ Drop into a squat position, placing your hands on the floor.

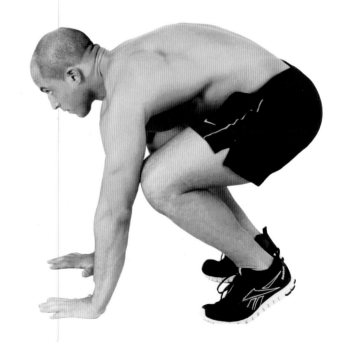

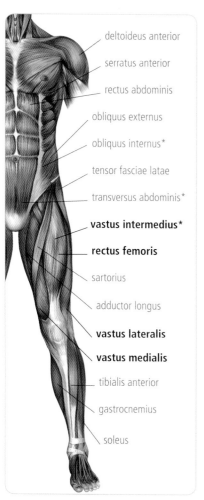

deltoideus anterior

serratus anterior

rectus abdominis

obliquus externus

obliquus internus*

tensor fasciae latae

transversus abdominis*

vastus intermedius*

rectus femoris

sartorius

adductor longus

vastus lateralis

vastus medialis

tibialis anterior

gastrocnemius

soleus

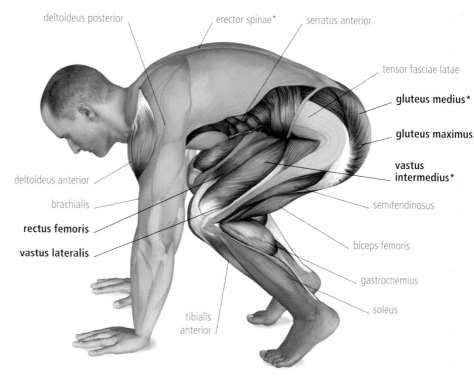

deltoideus posterior

erector spinae*

serratus anterior

tensor fasciae latae

gluteus medius*

gluteus maximus

vastus intermedius*

semitendinosus

biceps femoris

gastrocnemius

soleus

deltoideus anterior

brachialis

rectus femoris

vastus lateralis

tibialis anterior

BEST FOR

- **rectus femoris**
- **vastus lateralis**
- **vastus intermedius***
- **vastus medialis**
- **gluteus maximus**
- **gluteus medius***

ANNOTATION KEY

Bold text indicates target muscles

Grey text indicates other working muscles

* indicates deep muscles

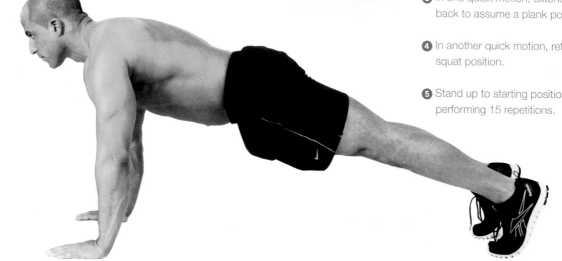

❸ In one quick motion, extend your feet back to assume a plank position.

❹ In another quick motion, return to the squat position.

❺ Stand up to starting position. Repeat, performing 15 repetitions.

MOUNTAIN CLIMBER

❶ Begin in an upper pushup position, palms and toes on the floor.

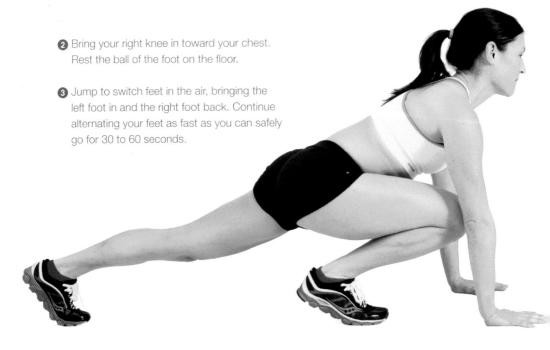

DO IT RIGHT
- As much as possible, keep your hands planted on the floor.
- Keep your shoulders pressed down.
- Maintain a quick pace.

AVOID
- Moving through the positions so quickly that you compromise your form.
- Hunching your shoulders.

BENEFITS
- Warms up muscles
- Improves coordination
- Strengthens and tones abdominal, chest, and leg muscles
- Plyometrically integrates explosive movement with cardiovascular exercise

PERFORMANCE BOOST
- All field sports

❷ Bring your right knee in toward your chest. Rest the ball of the foot on the floor.

❸ Jump to switch feet in the air, bringing the left foot in and the right foot back. Continue alternating your feet as fast as you can safely go for 30 to 60 seconds.

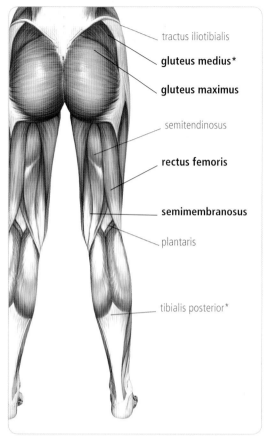

tractus iliotibialis

gluteus medius*

gluteus maximus

semitendinosus

rectus femoris

semimembranosus

plantaris

tibialis posterior*

ANNOTATION KEY

Bold text indicates target muscles

Grey text indicates other working muscles

* indicates deep muscles

BEST FOR

- **vastus lateralis**
- **rectus femoris**
- **gluteus maximus**
- **gluteus medius***
- **semimembranosus**
- **adductor magnus**
- **levator scapulae***
- **splenius***
- **trapezius**

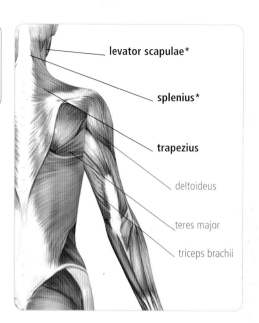

levator scapulae*

splenius*

trapezius

deltoideus

teres major

triceps brachii

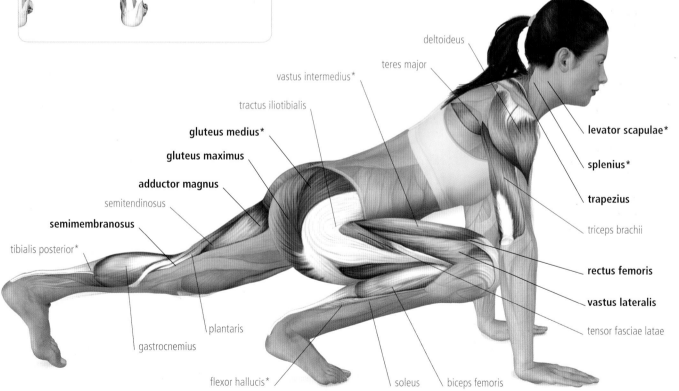

deltoideus

teres major

vastus intermedius*

tractus iliotibialis

gluteus medius*

gluteus maximus

adductor magnus

semitendinosus

semimembranosus

tibialis posterior*

plantaris

gastrocnemius

flexor hallucis*

soleus

biceps femoris

levator scapulae*

splenius*

trapezius

triceps brachii

rectus femoris

vastus lateralis

tensor fasciae latae

JUMPING LUNGE

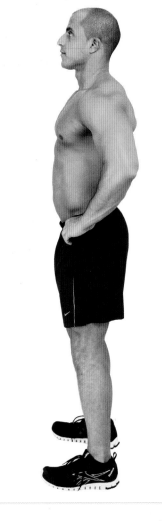

① Stand upright, with your feet hip-width apart and your hands on your hips.

AVOID
- Allowing your front knee to twist to either side.
- Hunching your shoulders.
- Tilting your torso.
- Arching your back.

DO IT RIGHT
- Keep breathing throughout the exercise.
- Keep your front knee facing forward.
- Keep your torso upright.
- Maintain a steady pace.
- Gaze forward.

BENEFITS
- Plyometrically integrates explosive movement with coordinated agility training

PERFORMANCE BOOST
- All field sports

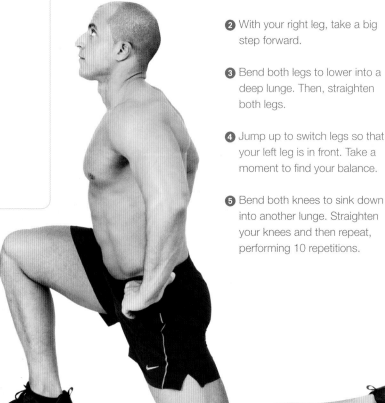

② With your right leg, take a big step forward.

③ Bend both legs to lower into a deep lunge. Then, straighten both legs.

④ Jump up to switch legs so that your left leg is in front. Take a moment to find your balance.

⑤ Bend both knees to sink down into another lunge. Straighten your knees and then repeat, performing 10 repetitions.

BEST FOR

- rectus femoris
- vastus lateralis
- vastus intermedius*
- vastus medialis
- biceps femoris
- semitendinosus
- semimembranosus
- gastrocnemius
- gluteus maximus
- gluteus medius*
- gluteus minimus*

ANNOTATION KEY

Bold text indicates target muscles

Grey text indicates other working muscles

* indicates deep muscles

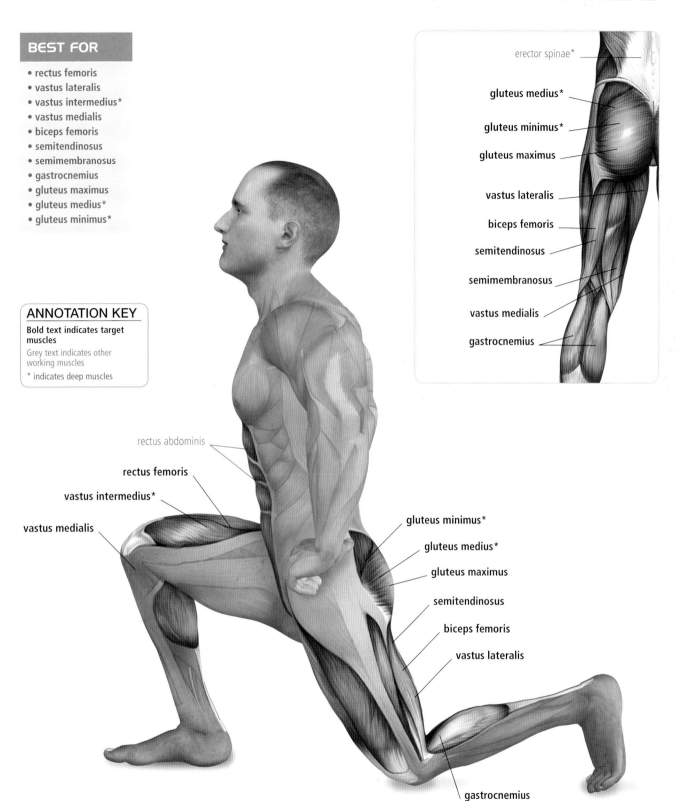

erector spinae*

gluteus medius*

gluteus minimus*

gluteus maximus

vastus lateralis

biceps femoris

semitendinosus

semimembranosus

vastus medialis

gastrocnemius

rectus abdominis

rectus femoris

vastus intermedius*

vastus medialis

gluteus minimus*

gluteus medius*

gluteus maximus

semitendinosus

biceps femoris

vastus lateralis

gastrocnemius

SWISS BALL JACKKNIFE

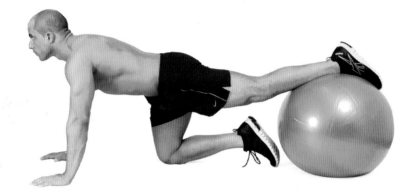

1 Kneel on your hands and knees, with the Swiss Ball behind you. Your hands should be planted on the floor, with your arms straight.

DO IT RIGHT
- Engage your core, keeping your abs pulled inward.
- Keep your back as straight as possible.
- Keep your body stable throughout.
- When your legs are extended n the ball, keep your legs, torso and neck in a straight line.
- Relax your neck.

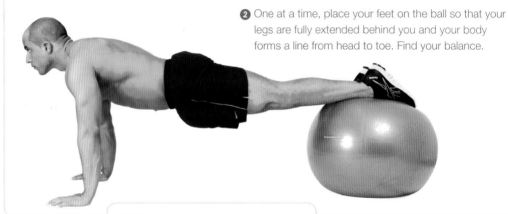

2 One at a time, place your feet on the ball so that your legs are fully extended behind you and your body forms a line from head to toe. Find your balance.

BENEFITS
- Improves coordination
- Strengthens core

PERFORMANCE BOOST
- All sports

AVOID
- Arching your back or neck.
- Letting your stomach bulge outward.

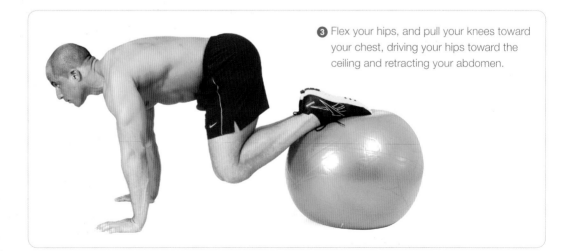

3 Flex your hips, and pull your knees toward your chest, driving your hips toward the ceiling and retracting your abdomen.

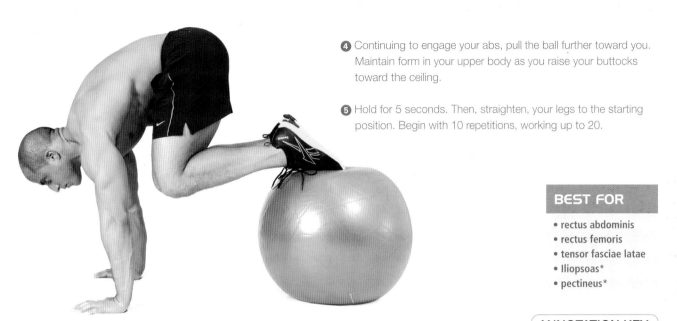

4 Continuing to engage your abs, pull the ball further toward you. Maintain form in your upper body as you raise your buttocks toward the ceiling.

5 Hold for 5 seconds. Then, straighten, your legs to the starting position. Begin with 10 repetitions, working up to 20.

BEST FOR

- **rectus abdominis**
- **rectus femoris**
- **tensor fasciae latae**
- **Iliopsoas***
- **pectineus***

ANNOTATION KEY

Bold text indicates target muscles

Grey text indicates other working muscles

* indicates deep muscles

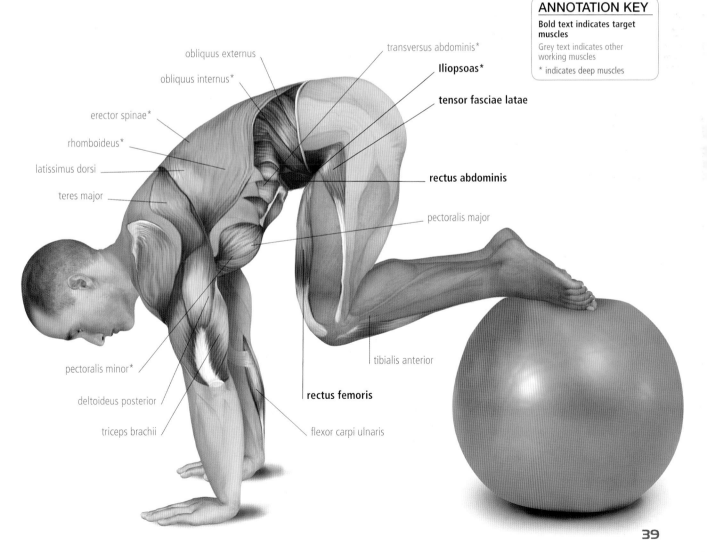

obliquus externus

obliquus internus*

erector spinae*

rhomboideus*

latissimus dorsi

teres major

pectoralis minor*

deltoideus posterior

triceps brachii

transversus abdominis*

Iliopsoas*

tensor fasciae latae

rectus abdominis

pectoralis major

tibialis anterior

rectus femoris

flexor carpi ulnaris

39

LEG-EXTENSION CHAIR DIP

1 Sit on the very edge of a chair, with your palms on the seat. Your back should be straight, your knees bent to form 90-degree angles.

2 Slowly and with control, engage your abdominal muscles and press your palms into the seat as you move your buttocks forward and lower slightly so that you are no longer resting on the chair.

AVOID
- Arching your back or hunching forward.
- Twisting your hips.

DO IT RIGHT
- Keep your supporting foot anchored to the floor.
- Keep your back straight.
- Keep your hips level.
- Gaze forward.

BENEFITS
- Improves balance
- Strengthens legs and triceps

PERFORMANCE BOOST
- All sports

3 Bending your arms slightly, extend your left leg forward to form a straight line.

4 Return your foot to the floor. Repeat on the other side, working up to 10 repetitions per side. Release and return to starting position.

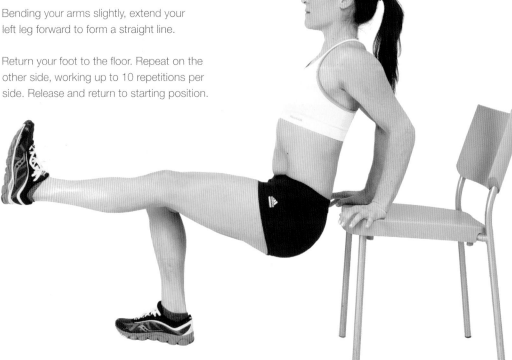

40

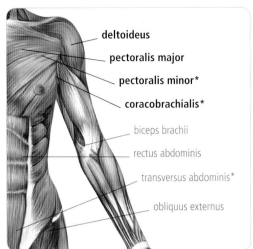

deltoideus

pectoralis major

pectoralis minor*

coracobrachialis*

biceps brachii

rectus abdominis

transversus abdominis*

obliquus externus

BEST FOR

- pectoralis major
- pectoralis minor*
- coracobrachialis*
- deltoideus
- deltoideus

ANNOTATION KEY

Bold text indicates target muscles

Grey text indicates other working muscles

* indicates deep muscles

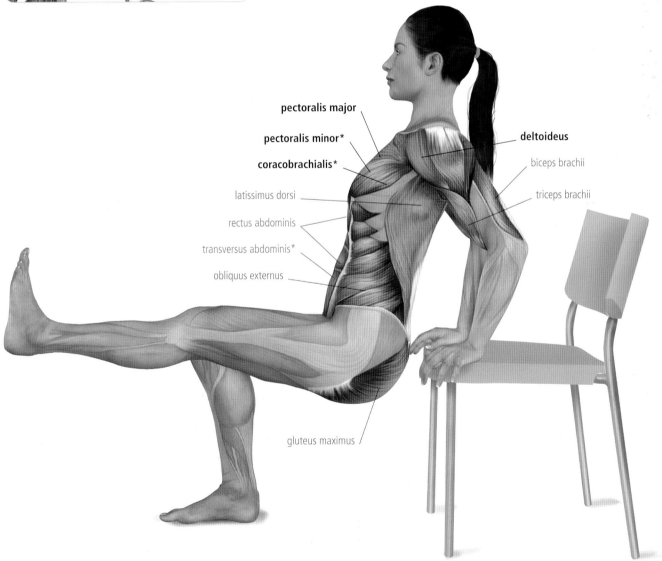

pectoralis major

pectoralis minor*

coracobrachialis*

latissimus dorsi

rectus abdominis

transversus abdominis*

obliquus externus

deltoideus

biceps brachii

triceps brachii

gluteus maximus

ONE-LEGGED STEP-DOWN

1 Stand facing forward on a step.

AVOID
- Allowing your knee to twist inward; instead, keep it in line with your middle toe.
- Rushing through the movement.

DO IT RIGHT
- Hold the wall or a rail for support if desired.
- Move slowly and with control.
- Focus on maintaining good form.

BENEFITS
- Strengthens pelvic and knee stabilisers

PERFORMANCE BOOST
- Running
- Rock-Climbing

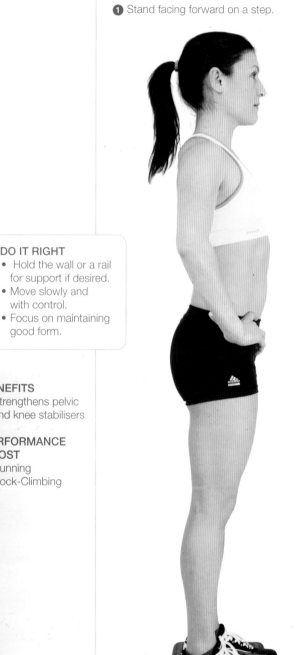

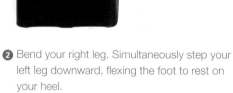

2 Bend your right leg. Simultaneously step your left leg downward, flexing the foot to rest on your heel.

3 Without rotating your torso or knee, press upward through your right leg to return to starting position. Switch legs and repeat, performing 20 repetitions.

BEST FOR

- deltoideus anterior
- quadratus lumborum*
- vastus lateralis
- vastus intermedius*
- vastus medialis
- sartorius
- rectus femoris
- gluteus maximus
- semitendinosus
- semimembranosus

ANNOTATION KEY

Bold text indicates target muscles

Grey text indicates other working muscles

* indicates deep muscles

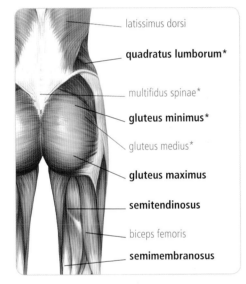

latissimus dorsi

quadratus lumborum*

multifidus spinae*

gluteus minimus*

gluteus medius*

gluteus maximus

semitendinosus

biceps femoris

semimembranosus

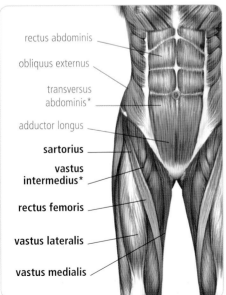

rectus abdominis

obliquus externus

transversus abdominis*

adductor longus

sartorius

vastus intermedius*

rectus femoris

vastus lateralis

vastus medialis

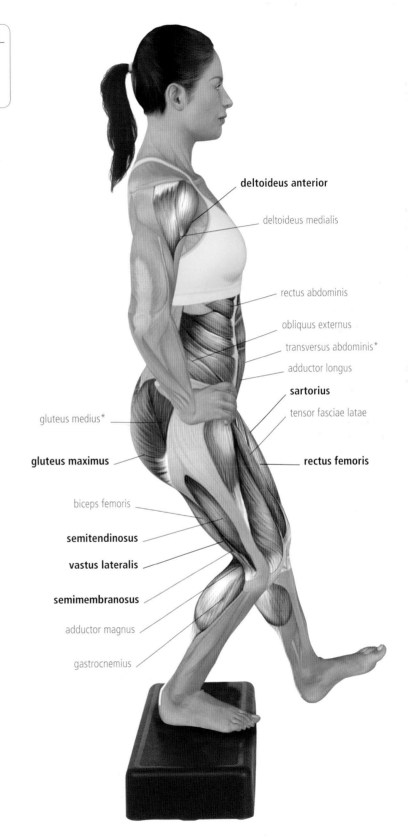

deltoideus anterior

deltoideus medialis

rectus abdominis

obliquus externus

transversus abdominis*

adductor longus

sartorius

tensor fasciae latae

rectus femoris

gluteus medius*

gluteus maximus

biceps femoris

semitendinosus

vastus lateralis

semimembranosus

adductor magnus

gastrocnemius

PUSH-UP WALKOUT

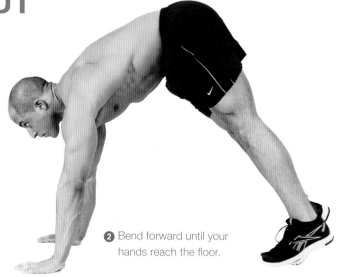

❶ Stand with your feet hip-width apart.

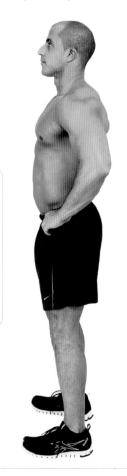

AVOID
- Arching your back or hunching forward.
- Going too far forward at first; instead, build up to the full walkout if desired.
- Tensing your neck.

BENEFITS
- Strengthens and tones core, chest and back muscles

PERFORMANCE BOOST
- All field sports

❷ Bend forward until your hands reach the floor.

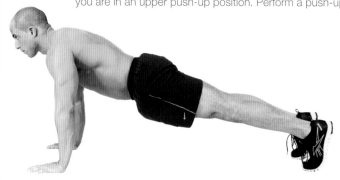

❸ 'Walk' your hands out in front of you as far as possible.

❹ Press your palms into the floor and tuck your toes so that you are in an upper push-up position. Perform a push-up.

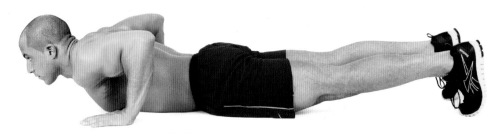

❺ 'Walk' the hands back toward your feet. Work up to 10 repetitions.

❻ Roll back up to starting position.

DO IT RIGHT
- Keep your feet planted on the floor as you 'walk' your hands forward and back.
- Keep your back in a neutral position while performing the push-up.
- Pull your stomach in and engage your abdominal muscles.

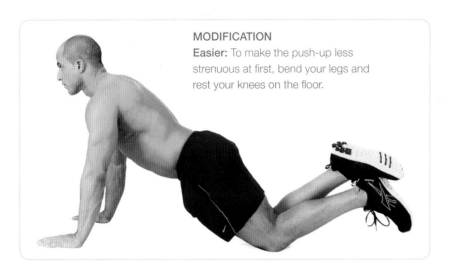

MODIFICATION
Easier: To make the push-up less strenuous at first, bend your legs and rest your knees on the floor.

BEST FOR

- rectus abdominis
- transversus abdominis*
- latissimus dorsi
- pectoralis major
- brachialis
- coracobrachialis*
- pectoralis minor*
- deltoideus anterior

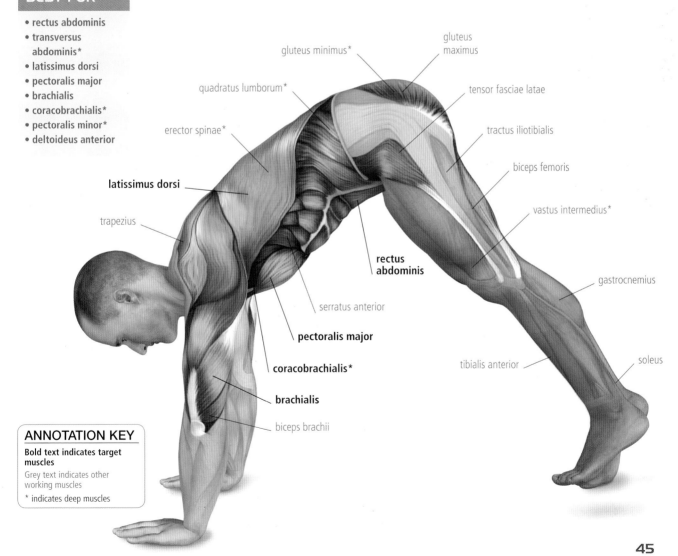

gluteus minimus*

gluteus maximus

quadratus lumborum*

tensor fasciae latae

erector spinae*

tractus iliotibialis

latissimus dorsi

biceps femoris

trapezius

vastus intermedius*

rectus abdominis

gastrocnemius

serratus anterior

pectoralis major

coracobrachialis*

tibialis anterior

soleus

brachialis

biceps brachii

ANNOTATION KEY
Bold text indicates target muscles

Grey text indicates other working muscles

* indicates deep muscles

ARM-REACH PLANK

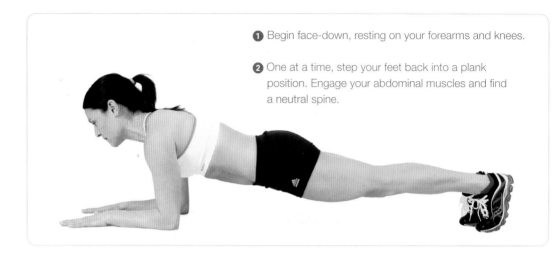

❶ Begin face-down, resting on your forearms and knees.

❷ One at a time, step your feet back into a plank position. Engage your abdominal muscles and find a neutral spine.

BENEFITS
- Improves balance
- Strengthens and tones arms, legs and abdominal muscles

PERFORMANCE BOOST
- Swimming
- Gymnastics
- Dance

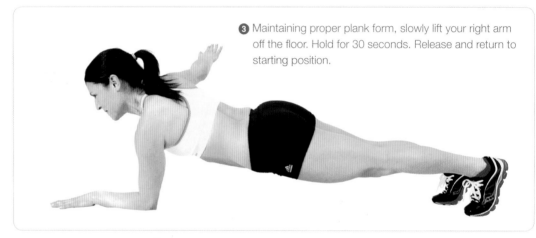

❸ Maintaining proper plank form, slowly lift your right arm off the floor. Hold for 30 seconds. Release and return to starting position.

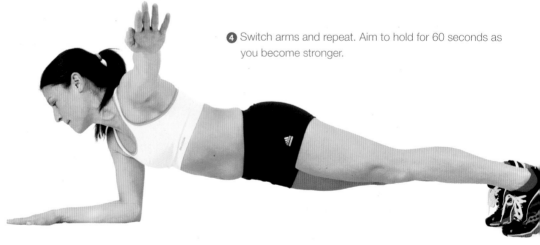

❹ Switch arms and repeat. Aim to hold for 60 seconds as you become stronger.

AVOID
- Allowing your hips to sink or tilt upward.
- Letting your abs bulge outward.

DO IT RIGHT
- Contract your abdominal muscles.
- Keep your spine parallel to the floor.

MODIFICATION

Easier: Instead of raising each arm fully off the floor, lift only your forearm. Additionally, try bending your knees to make the exercise less strenuous.

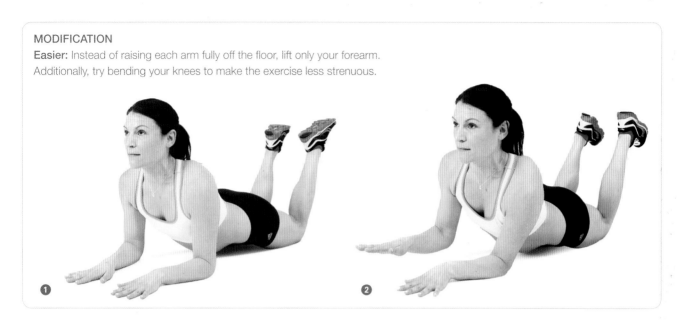

ANNOTATION KEY

Bold text indicates target muscles

Grey text indicates other working muscles

* indicates deep muscles

BEST FOR

- brachioradialis
- brachialis
- latissimus dorsi
- rectus abdominis
- obliquus externus
- tractus iliotibialis
- rectus femoris

latissimus dorsi

obliquus externus

obliquus internus*

tractus iliotibialis

tensor fasciae latae

pectineus*

adductor longus

soleus

deltoideus

biceps brachii

flexor digitorum*

rectus abdominis

transversus abdominis*

brachialis

gracilis*

brachioradialis

rectus femoris

tibialis anterior

peroneus

vastus medialis

extensor digitorum

TWISTING KNEE RAISE

1 Stand with your feet hip-width apart and your arms at your sides. Raise both arms and bend your elbows so that each arm forms a right angle, palms facing forward.

2 Raise your left knee toward your abdomen. At the same time, bring your right elbow toward the knee. Aim for your knee and elbow to touch.

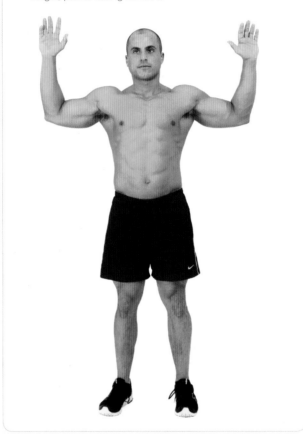

BENEFITS
• Improves balance and coordination
• Strengthens and tones core muscles and calves

PERFORMANCE BOOST
• Football
• All field sports

AVOID
• Hyperextending your back.
• Letting your hips twist excessively.

DO IT RIGHT
• Keep your abs engaged and contracted.
• Maintain a quick pace.
• Face forward as you perform the twist.

3 Return to starting position. Repeat, alternating sides. Aim for 20 repetitions.

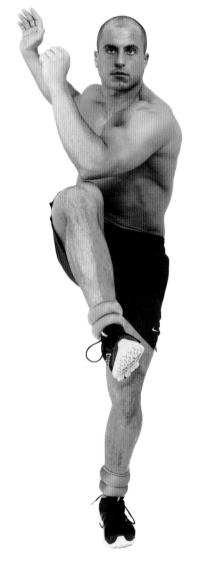

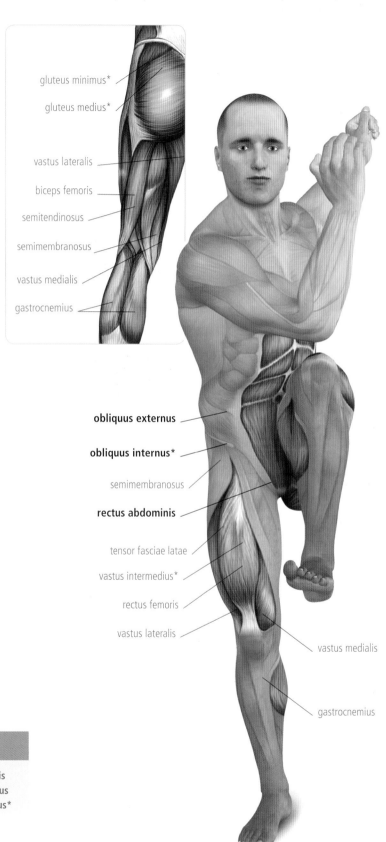

gluteus minimus*

gluteus medius*

vastus lateralis

biceps femoris

semitendinosus

semimembranosus

vastus medialis

gastrocnemius

obliquus externus

obliquus internus*

semimembranosus

rectus abdominis

tensor fasciae latae

vastus intermedius*

rectus femoris

vastus lateralis

vastus medialis

gastrocnemius

ANNOTATION KEY

Bold text indicates target muscles

Grey text indicates other working muscles

* indicates deep muscles

BEST FOR

- **rectus abdominis**
- **obliquus externus**
- **obliquus internus***

HEEL BEAT

❶ Lie facedown with your forearms on the floor. Rest your hips on top of a small Swiss ball. Extend your legs behind you.

❷ Turn your legs out from the top of your hips.

AVOID
• Hunching your shoulders.
• Tensing your neck.

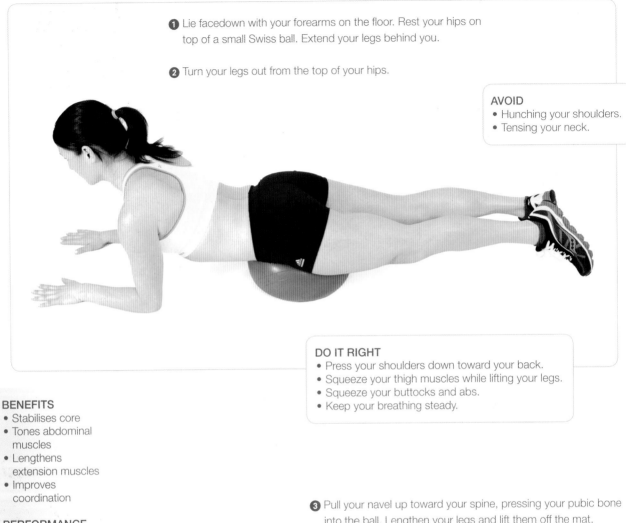

DO IT RIGHT
• Press your shoulders down toward your back.
• Squeeze your thigh muscles while lifting your legs.
• Squeeze your buttocks and abs.
• Keep your breathing steady.

BENEFITS
• Stabilises core
• Tones abdominal muscles
• Lengthens extension muscles
• Improves coordination

PERFORMANCE BOOST
• Swimming
• All field sports

❸ Pull your navel up toward your spine, pressing your pubic bone into the ball. Lengthen your legs and lift them off the mat.

❹ Press your heels together and then separate them in a rapid but controlled motion.

❺ Beat your heels together for 8 counts. Release and then repeat, performing 6 repetitions.

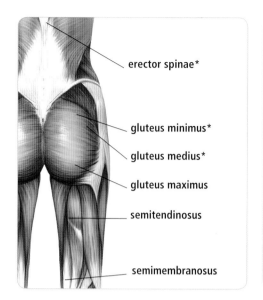

erector spinae*

gluteus minimus*

gluteus medius*

gluteus maximus

semitendinosus

semimembranosus

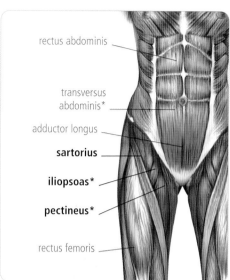

rectus abdominis

transversus abdominis*

adductor longus

sartorius

iliopsoas*

pectineus*

rectus femoris

BEST FOR

- gluteus maximus
- gluteus medius*
- gluteus minimus*
- erector spinae*
- sartorius
- pectineus*
- iliopsoas*

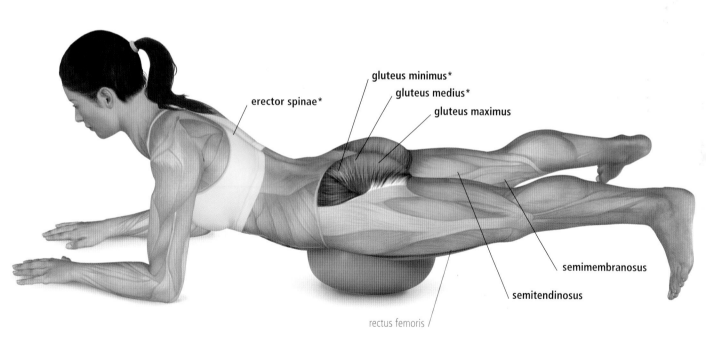

erector spinae*

gluteus minimus*

gluteus medius*

gluteus maximus

semimembranosus

semitendinosus

rectus femoris

ANNOTATION KEY

Bold text indicates target muscles

Grey text indicates other working muscles

* indicates deep muscles

SWIMMING

1 Lie on your stomach with your legs hip-width apart. Stretch your arms beside your ears on the floor. Engage your pelvic floor, and draw your navel into your spine.

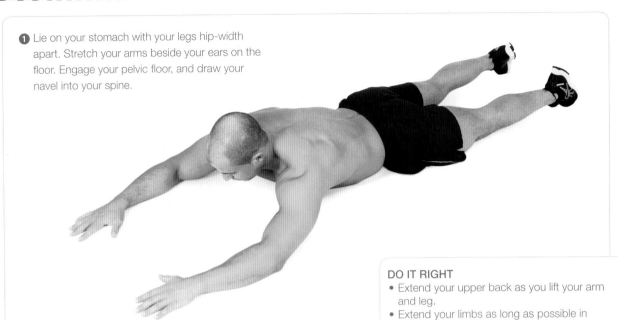

DO IT RIGHT
- Extend your upper back as you lift your arm and leg.
- Extend your limbs as long as possible in opposite directions.
- Keep your glutes tightly squeezed.
- Draw your navel toward your spine.
- Press your shoulders down toward your back.
- Keep your resting arm and leg on the floor.
- Relax your neck.

BENEFITS
- Stabilises core
- Tones abdominal muscles
- Strengthens hip and spinal extensors
- Challenges stabilisation of the spine against rotation

PERFORMANCE BOOST
- Swimming
- All field sports

2 Lift your right arm and left leg simultaneously. Raise your head slightly off the floor.

3 Lower your arm and leg to the starting position, maintaining a stretch in your limbs.

4 Repeat on the other side. Aim for 8 repetitions.

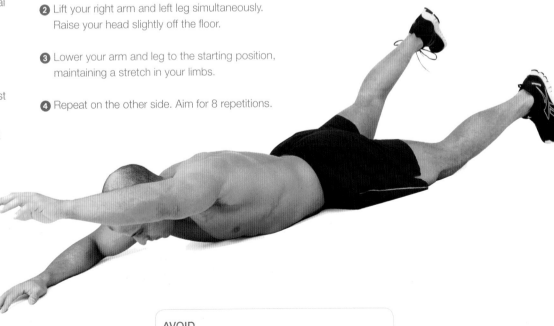

AVOID
- Tensing your neck.
- Lifting your shoulders toward your ears.

MODIFICATION

Harder: Lift your arms and legs at the same time, and move them as if you were making snow angels. Keep your abs engaged and your back neutral as you move.

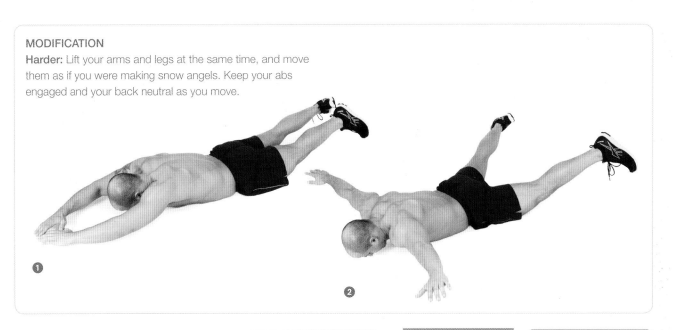

1

2

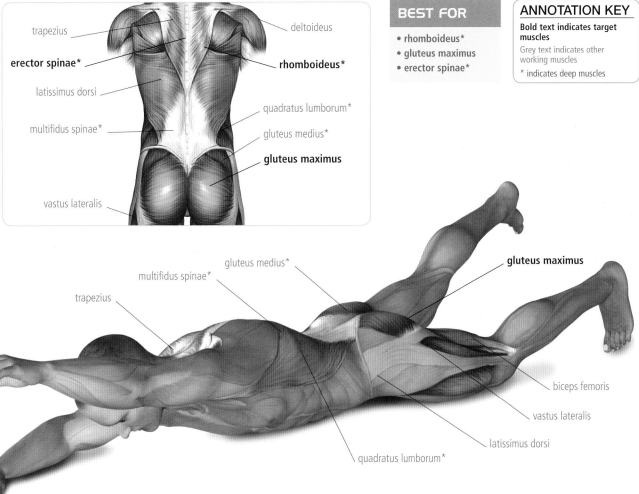

trapezius

deltoideus

erector spinae*

rhomboideus*

latissimus dorsi

multifidus spinae*

quadratus lumborum*

gluteus medius*

gluteus maximus

vastus lateralis

gluteus medius*

multifidus spinae*

trapezius

gluteus maximus

biceps femoris

vastus lateralis

latissimus dorsi

quadratus lumborum*

PIRIFORMIS BRIDGE

1 Lie on your back, arms extended at your sides. Your knees should be bent, with feet on the floor.

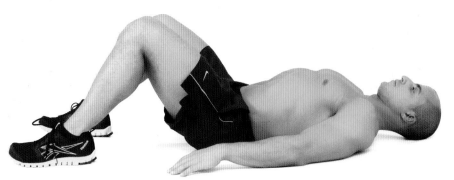

2 Keeping the rest of your body still, raise your left leg to rest the ankle on your right knee.

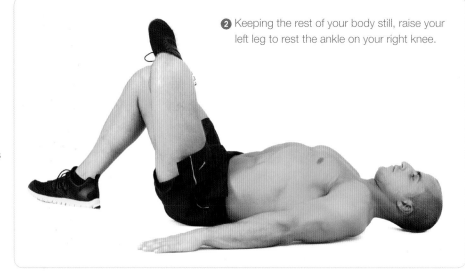

BENEFITS
• Stretches piriformis
• Strengthens quadriceps, hamstrings and gluteal muscles
• Stabilizes core

PERFORMANCE BOOST
• Rollerblading and skating
• All field sports

DO IT RIGHT
• Squeeze your buttocks as you lift and lower.
• Draw your navel toward your spine.
• Press your shoulders down toward your back.
• Anchor your arms to the floor.
• Relax your neck.

AVOID
• Tensing your neck.
• Lifting your shoulders toward your ears.

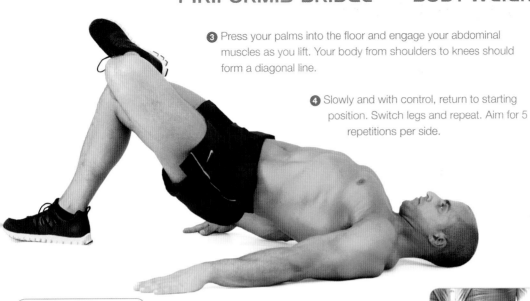

3 Press your palms into the floor and engage your abdominal muscles as you lift. Your body from shoulders to knees should form a diagonal line.

4 Slowly and with control, return to starting position. Switch legs and repeat. Aim for 5 repetitions per side.

BEST FOR

- **gluteus maximus**
- **gluteus medius***
- **gluteus minimus***
- **biceps femoris**
- **semitendinosus**
- **semimembranosus**
- **rectus femoris**
- **vastus lateralis**
- **vastus intermedius***
- **vastus medialis**

ANNOTATION KEY

Bold text indicates target muscles

Grey text indicates other working muscles

* indicates deep muscles

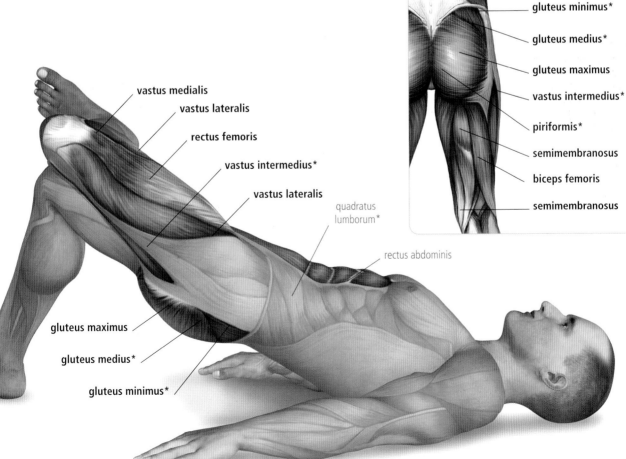

vastus medialis
vastus lateralis
rectus femoris
vastus intermedius*
vastus lateralis
quadratus lumborum*
rectus abdominis
gluteus maximus
gluteus medius*
gluteus minimus*

erector spinae*
multifidus spinae*
quadratus lumborum*
gluteus minimus*
gluteus medius*
gluteus maximus
vastus intermedius*
piriformis*
semimembranosus
biceps femoris
semimembranosus

SWISS BALL BRIDGING RAISE

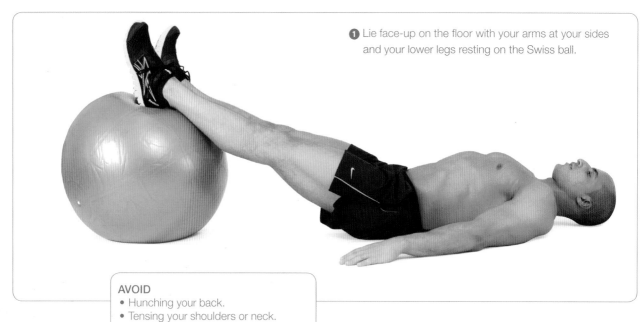

1 Lie face-up on the floor with your arms at your sides and your lower legs resting on the Swiss ball.

AVOID
- Hunching your back.
- Tensing your shoulders or neck.
- Letting the Swiss ball wobble.

DO IT RIGHT
- Keep your back in a neutral position.
- Press your shoulders down your back.
- Engage your abdominal muscles.

BENEFITS
- Stabilises pelvis and core
- Strengthens gluteal muscles and hamstrings

PERFORMANCE BOOST
- All field sports

2 Press your palms into the floor and engage your abdominal muscles as you lift your upper body off the floor. Your body should form a diagonal line. If desired, hold for a few seconds.

3 Slowly and with control, lower back to starting position. Repeat, performing 10 repetitions.

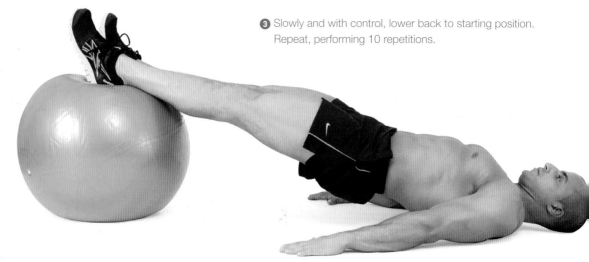

SWISS BALL BRIDGING RAISE • BODY-WEIGHT EXERCISES

BEST FOR

- biceps femoris
- semitendinosus
- semimembranosus

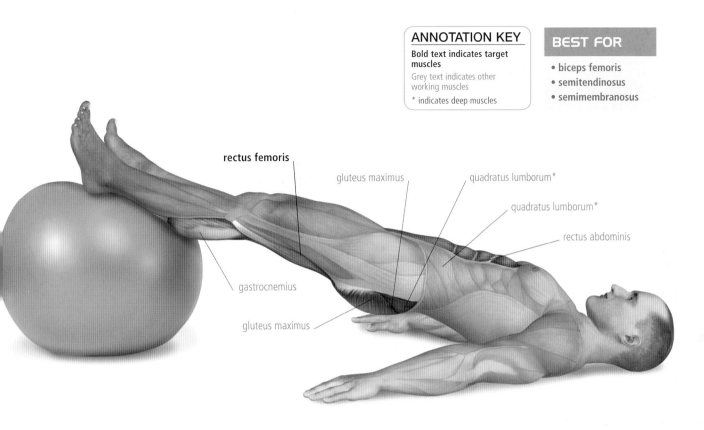

rectus femoris

gluteus maximus

quadratus lumborum*

quadratus lumborum*

rectus abdominis

gastrocnemius

gluteus maximus

MODIFICATION

Harder: In the raised position, lift one leg off the ball, extending it upward while maintaining your form. Return to starting position. Repeat on the other side, keeping both legs straight and your back neutral as you move.

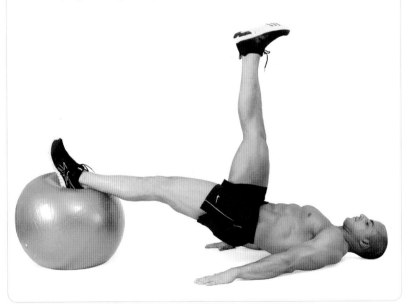

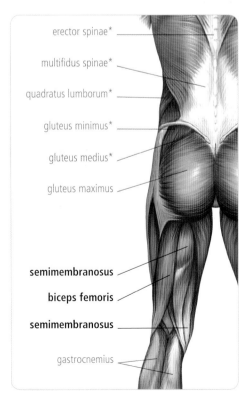

erector spinae*

multifidus spinae*

quadratus lumborum*

gluteus minimus*

gluteus medius*

gluteus maximus

semimembranosus

biceps femoris

semimembranosus

gastrocnemius

CHIN-UP WITH HANGING LEG RAISE

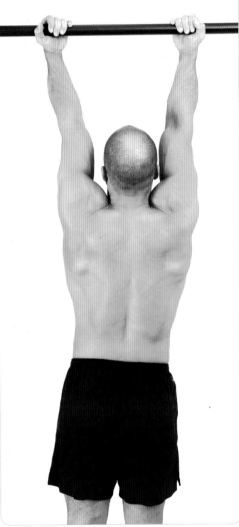

1 Begin hanging from a chin-up bar, gripping it firmly with both hands.

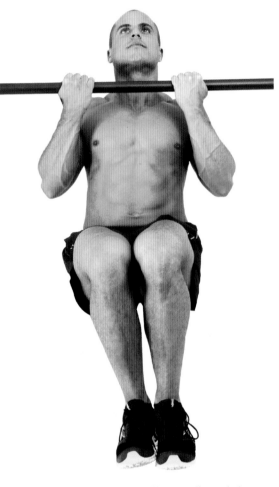

BENEFITS
• Strengthens arms and core

PERFORMANCE BOOST
• Gymnastics
• Tennis
• Football
• Baseball

2 Use your arm muscles to lift yourself up, aiming to bring your chin over the bar.

3 With your abdominal muscles strongly engaged, raise your knees. Hold for as long as possible.

4 Slowly straighten your legs. Then, straighten your arms as you return to starting position.

DO IT RIGHT
• Keep your feet together as you raise your knees.
• Keep your movement slow and controlled.
• Engage your core muscles throughout this challenging exercise.

AVOID
• Moving in a jerky manner.
• Arching your back.
• Tensing your neck.

ANNOTATION KEY

Bold text indicates target muscles

Grey text indicates other working muscles

* indicates deep muscles

BEST FOR

- latissimus dorsi
- rectus abdominis
- obliquus externus
- transversus abdominis*
- obliquus internus*
- serratus anterior
- triceps brachii

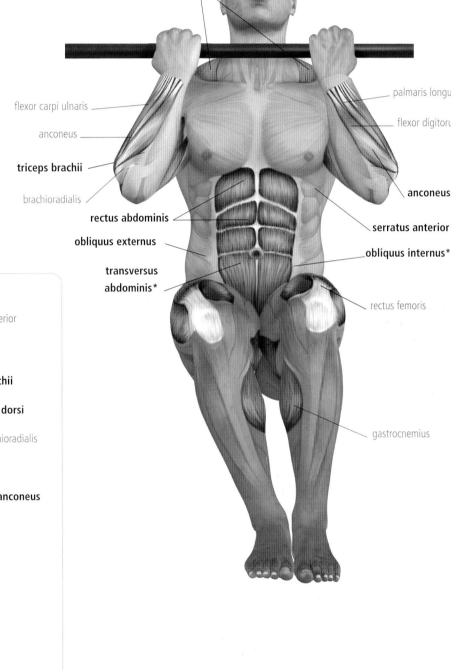

trapezius

flexor carpi ulnaris

anconeus

triceps brachii

brachioradialis

rectus abdominis

obliquus externus

transversus abdominis*

palmaris longus

flexor digitorum*

anconeus

serratus anterior

obliquus internus*

rectus femoris

gastrocnemius

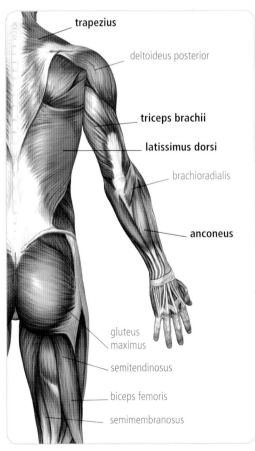

trapezius

deltoideus posterior

triceps brachii

latissimus dorsi

brachioradialis

anconeus

gluteus maximus

semitendinosus

biceps femoris

semimembranosus

FULL-BODY ROLL

❶ Lie on your back, with your arms extended at your sides and your legs extended on the floor.

❷ Raise your right leg so that it is perpendicular to the floor.

DO IT RIGHT
- Keep your abdominal muscles, especially your obliques, engaged as you roll.
- Keep your legs straight.
- Move at a steady pace

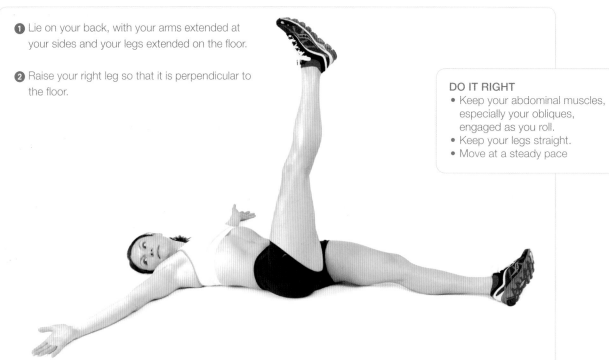

BENEFITS
- Tones cores muscles, especially obliques

PERFORMANCE BOOST
- All sports

❸ Lower your right leg toward the floor and then use your abdominal muscles and arms to roll to the left until you are face-down.

❹ Straighten your arms, lifting your upper torso off the ground. Your legs should be extended behind you.

❺ Roll onto your back, legs and arms extended in starting position. Then, raise your left leg and repeat the roll in the other direction. Repeat, alternating sides for 8 repetitions.

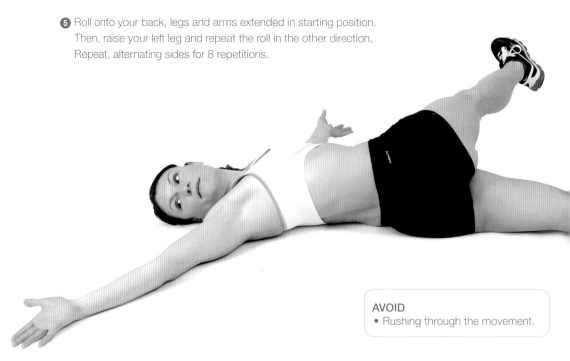

AVOID
- Rushing through the movement.

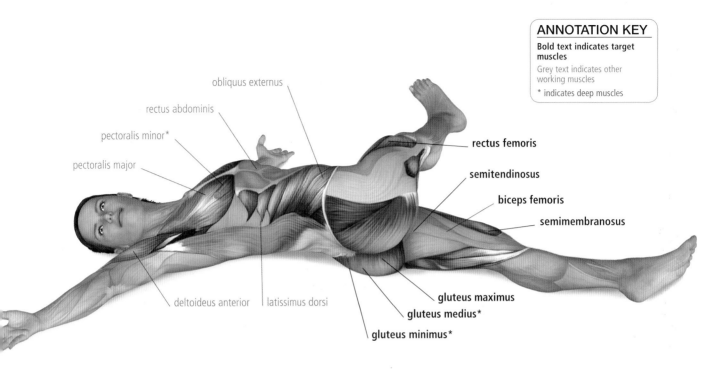

ANNOTATION KEY

Bold text indicates target muscles

Grey text indicates other working muscles

* indicates deep muscles

obliquus externus

rectus abdominis

pectoralis minor*

pectoralis major

rectus femoris

semitendinosus

biceps femoris

semimembranosus

deltoideus anterior | latissimus dorsi

gluteus maximus

gluteus medius*

gluteus minimus*

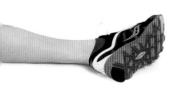

BEST FOR

- **vastus lateralis**
- **vastus intermedius***
- **vastus medialis**
- **rectus femoris**
- **iliopsoas***
- **biceps femoris**
- **semitendinosus**
- **semimembranosus**
- **gluteus maximus**
- **gluteus medius***
- **gluteus minimus***

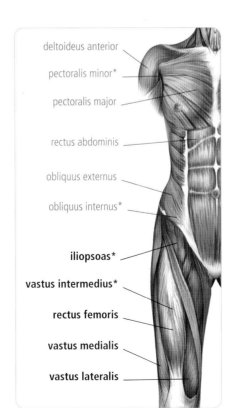

deltoideus anterior

pectoralis minor*

pectoralis major

rectus abdominis

obliquus externus

obliquus internus*

iliopsoas*

vastus intermedius*

rectus femoris

vastus medialis

vastus lateralis

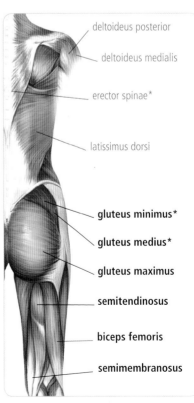

deltoideus posterior

deltoideus medialis

erector spinae*

latissimus dorsi

gluteus minimus*

gluteus medius*

gluteus maximus

semitendinosus

biceps femoris

semimembranosus

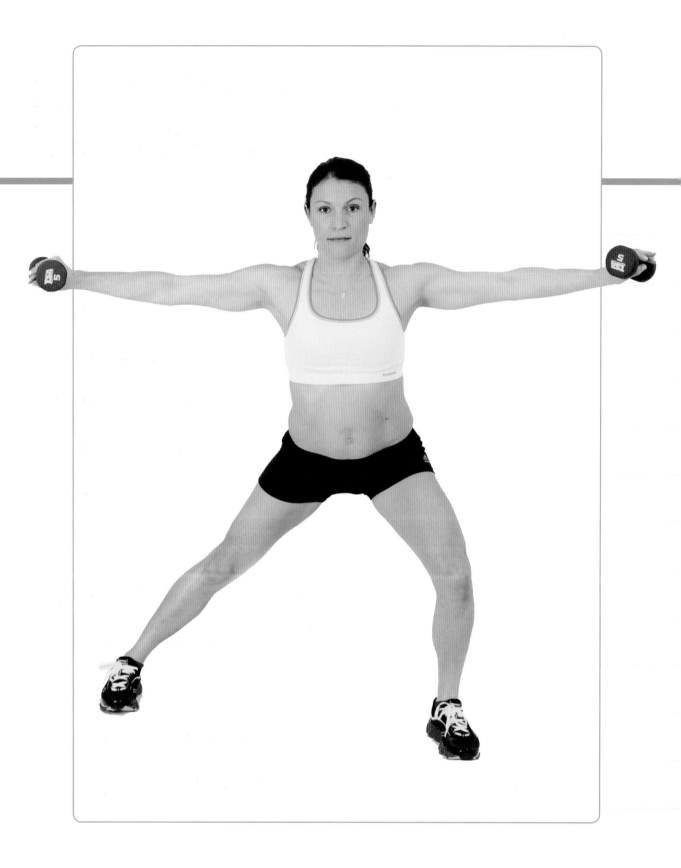

ADDED-WEIGHT EXERCISES

In the weight room, functional training takes an unusual route to fitness, eschewing the 'exercise to fatigue' adage in favour of, well, mixing it up. If you notice your previously pristine form suffering – your hips twisting to one side during Knee Raise with Lateral Extension, or your back arching while you hold Dead Lift – then don't power through. Instead, pause, turn the page, perhaps swap your barbells for a body bar, change position, and perform another exercise before returning to the Dead Lift, which you'll now approach with better form. Zoom through a zillion repetitions and you'll miss out on the good stuff: the spinal integrity, core stability, muscle engagement, balance, and dynamism that will help you excel at any of life's challenges.

REACH-AND-TWIST WALKING LUNGE

1 Stand with feet roughly hip-width apart and your torso facing forward. Hold a weighted medicine ball in both hands.

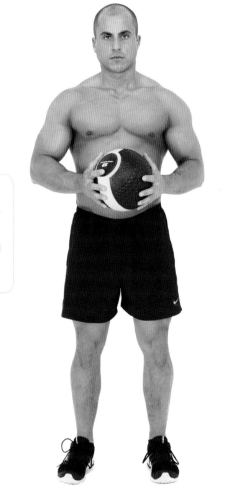

2 Lunge your left foot forward. Begin to bend both knees, lowering your whole body into the lunge. At the same time, raise the medicine ball until it is over your left shoulder, held in both hands.

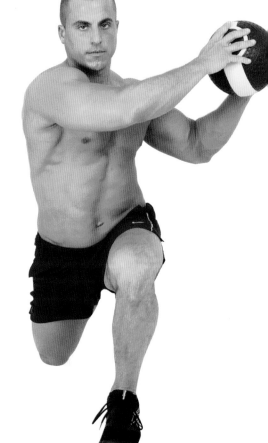

DO IT RIGHT
- As much as possible, keep your torso facing forward.
- Keep your abdominal muscles engaged.
- Move smoothly.

BENEFITS
- Builds endurance and coordination
- Strengthens and tones core, especially abdominal and gluteal muscles

PERFORMANCE BOOST
- Football
- Baseball
- Tennis
- Squash

AVOID
- Hunching your shoulders.
- Arching your back.
- Turning your neck in either direction.
- Letting your belly bulge outward.
- Losing control of the medicine ball.
- Letting the medicine ball be held more by one hand than the other.

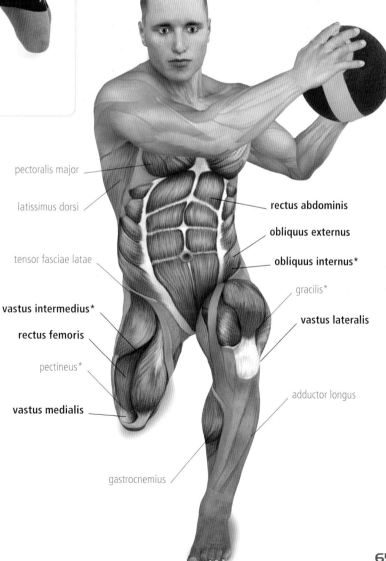

BEST FOR

- rectus femoris
- vastus lateralis
- vastus intermedius*
- vastus medialis
- gluteus maximus
- biceps femoris
- semitendinosus
- semimembranosus
- rectus abdominis
- obliquus externus
- obliquus internus*

ANNOTATION KEY

Bold text indicates target muscles

Grey text indicates other working muscles

* indicates deep muscles

❸ In a single motion, rise up to stand, bring the ball back to centre, and then perform the lunge and reach in the other direction.

❹ Continue to lunge and move the ball from side to side as you walk forward. Continue for 15 steps.

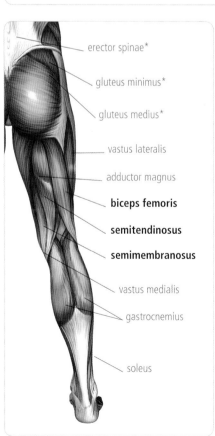

erector spinae*

gluteus minimus*

gluteus medius*

vastus lateralis

adductor magnus

biceps femoris

semitendinosus

semimembranosus

vastus medialis

gastrocnemius

soleus

pectoralis major

latissimus dorsi

tensor fasciae latae

vastus intermedius*

rectus femoris

pectineus*

vastus medialis

gastrocnemius

rectus abdominis

obliquus externus

obliquus internus*

gracilis*

vastus lateralis

adductor longus

CLEAN-AND-PRESS

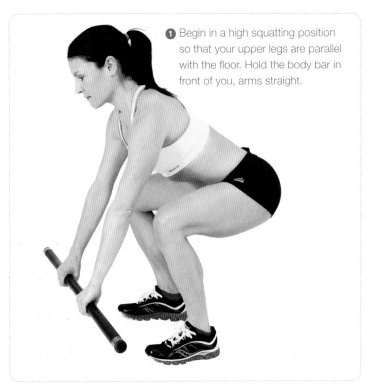

1 Begin in a high squatting position so that your upper legs are parallel with the floor. Hold the body bar in front of you, arms straight.

DO IT RIGHT
- Your back should be in a neutral S-curve position during all steps of the exercises.
- Engage your legs and core muscles as you rise to stand.
- While you raise the bar overhead, keep your abdominals strongly engaged.

2 Using the muscles in your legs as well as your abdominals, rise to stand as you bend your arms to bring the bar to shoulder height. If you choose, extend one foot in front of the other.

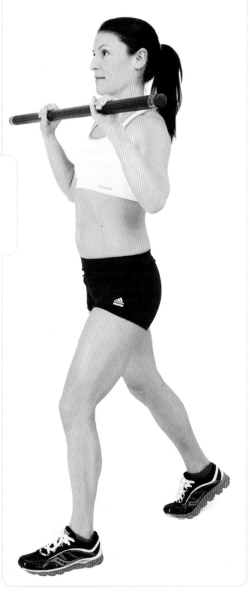

BENEFITS
- Strengthens and tones whole body

PERFORMANCE BOOST
- Tennis
- Volleyball
- All field sports

AVOID
- Hunching your shoulders.
- Letting your abdominals bulge outward.
- Distorting the S-curve of your spine by arching your back or hunching forward.
- Rushing through the movement.

CLEAN-AND-PRESS • ADDED-WEIGHT EXERCISES

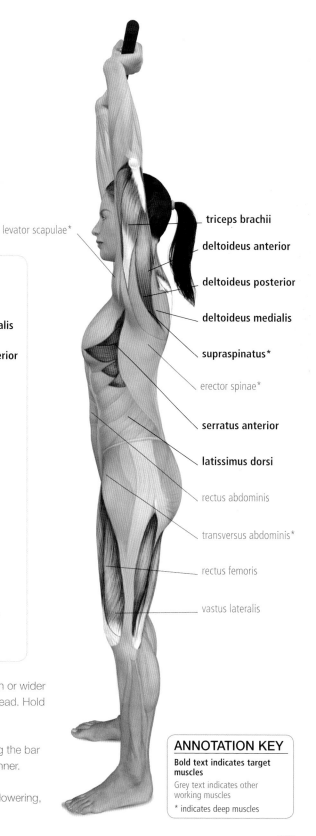

BEST FOR

- latissimus dorsi
- trapezius
- deltoideus anterior
- deltoideus posterior
- deltoideus medialis
- triceps brachii
- serratus anterior
- supraspinatus*

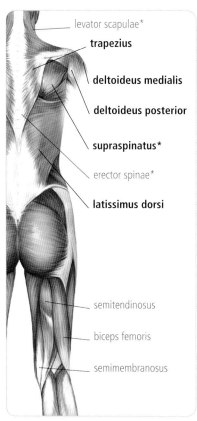

levator scapulae*

trapezius

deltoideus medialis

deltoideus posterior

supraspinatus*

erector spinae*

latissimus dorsi

semitendinosus

biceps femoris

semimembranosus

levator scapulae*

triceps brachii

deltoideus anterior

deltoideus posterior

deltoideus medialis

supraspinatus*

erector spinae*

serratus anterior

latissimus dorsi

rectus abdominis

transversus abdominis*

rectus femoris

vastus lateralis

❸ Move your feet to parallel position, hip-width or wider apart, and bring the body bar above your head. Hold for several seconds.

❹ Focus on breath and alignment as you bring the bar down to shoulder height in a controlled manner.

❺ Repeat the lift overhead and the controlled lowering, aiming for 10 repetitions.

ANNOTATION KEY

Bold text indicates target muscles

Grey text indicates other working muscles

* indicates deep muscles

KNEE-FLEXION BALL THROW

① Hold a weighted medicine ball in front of your chest, taking a few steps forward to get ready if you choose.

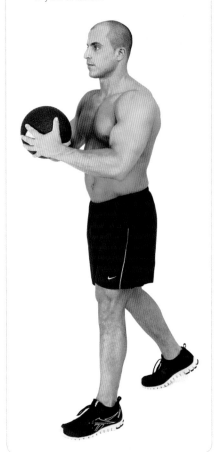

② Prepare to throw the ball by positioning your left foot behind you, heel off the floor. Keeping your torso stable, raise the ball until it is positioned above your right shoulder.

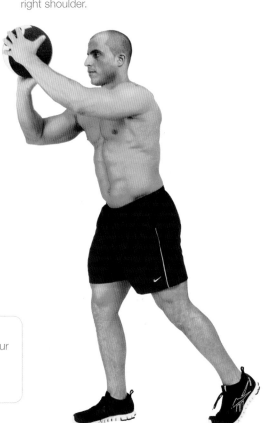

BENEFITS
- Improves coordination, core rotational ability and range of motion in upper body
- Strengthens and stabilises core

PERFORMANCE BOOST
- Basketball
- Football
- Tennis
- Squash

AVOID
- Excessively twisting your torso to either side.
- Hunching your shoulders.

DO IT RIGHT
- Gaze forward.
- Keep your torso facing forward.
- Engage your abdominal muscles as you throw.

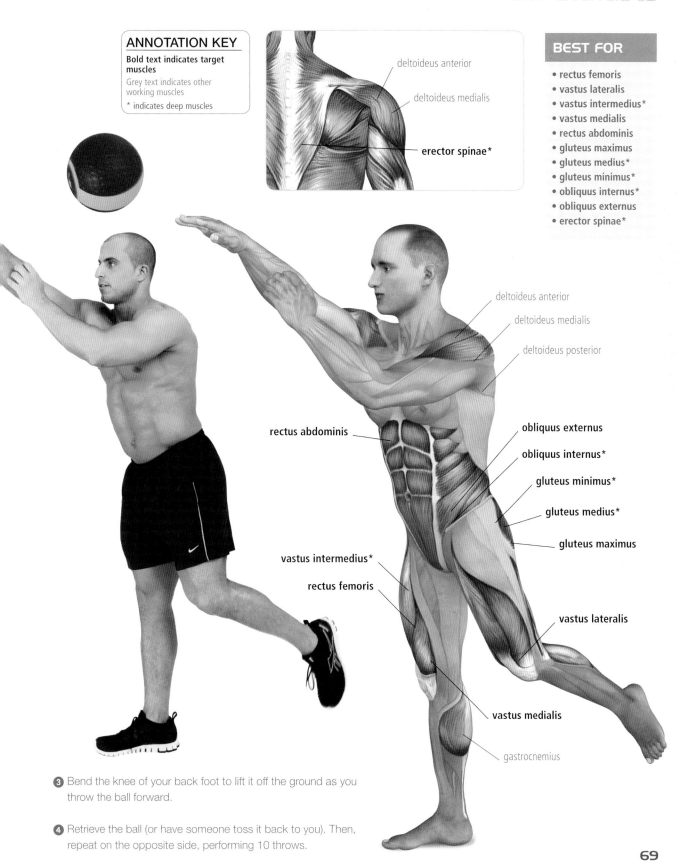

ANNOTATION KEY

Bold text indicates target muscles

Grey text indicates other working muscles

* indicates deep muscles

deltoideus anterior

deltoideus medialis

erector spinae*

BEST FOR

- **rectus femoris**
- **vastus lateralis**
- **vastus intermedius***
- **vastus medialis**
- **rectus abdominis**
- **gluteus maximus**
- **gluteus medius***
- **gluteus minimus***
- **obliquus internus***
- **obliquus externus**
- **erector spinae***

deltoideus anterior

deltoideus medialis

deltoideus posterior

rectus abdominis

obliquus externus

obliquus internus*

gluteus minimus*

gluteus medius*

gluteus maximus

vastus intermedius*

rectus femoris

vastus lateralis

vastus medialis

gastrocnemius

❸ Bend the knee of your back foot to lift it off the ground as you throw the ball forward.

❹ Retrieve the ball (or have someone toss it back to you). Then, repeat on the opposite side, performing 10 throws.

HEEL RAISE WITH OVERHEAD PRESS

❶ Stand with your feet hip-width apart and your arms at your sides, a dumbbell in each hand.

❷ Raise your arms, bending your elbows and lifting until the dumbbells are at ear height.

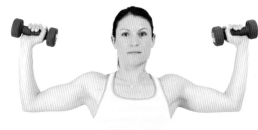
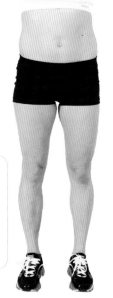
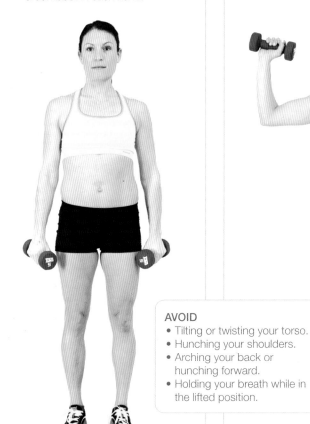
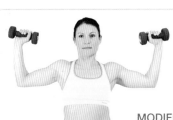
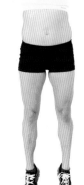

BENEFITS
• Strengthens and tones shoulders and calves

PERFORMANCE BOOST
• Tennis
• Volleyball
• Squash
• All field sports

AVOID
• Tilting or twisting your torso.
• Hunching your shoulders.
• Arching your back or hunching forward.
• Holding your breath while in the lifted position.

MODIFICATION
Easier: Bring your arms to ear level only as you raise your heels. Try holding for a few seconds before you release.

DO IT RIGHT
• Keep your torso facing forward.
• Pull your abdominal muscles inward.
• Raise and lower your arms smoothly and with control.
• Gaze forward.
• Keep your back in a neutral position, envisioning your spine lengthening as you lift your heels.
• Use your core muscles to help you balance while heels are lifted.

3 Bring your weights overhead as you lift your heels off the floor to stand on your tiptoes. Balance for a few seconds, if desired.

4 Lower your heels to the floor and bring your arms back to starting position. Repeat, aiming for 15 repetitions with good form.

BEST FOR

- gastrocnemius
- latissimus dorsi
- deltoideus anterior

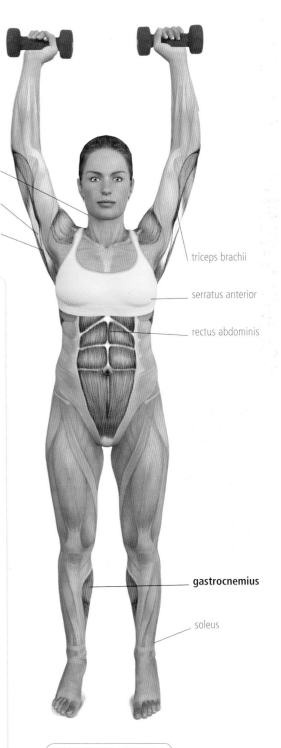

levator scapulae*

deltoideus medialis

deltoideus posterior

triceps brachii

serratus anterior

rectus abdominis

gastrocnemius

soleus

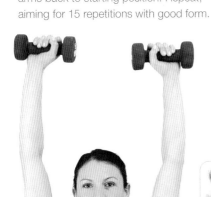

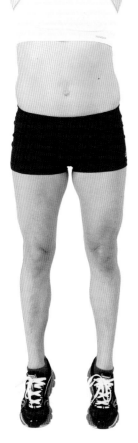

levator scapulae*

supraspinatus*

trapezius

deltoideus posterior

deltoideus anterior

deltoideus medialis

teres major

rhomboideus*

erector spinae*

latissimus dorsi

gluteus minimus*

gastrocnemius

soleus

ANNOTATION KEY

Bold text indicates target muscles

Grey text indicates other working muscles

* indicates deep muscles

LATERAL-EXTENSION LATERAL LUNGE

1 Stand with your feet hip-width apart and your arms at your sides, a dumbbell in each hand.

AVOID
- Positioning one arm in front of the other in the raised position.
- Hunching your shoulders.
- Arching your back or hunching forward.
- Twisting your torso to either side.

2 Take a big step to the left, and then bend your left knee to assume a side lunge position. At the same time, raise both arms so that they are parallel to the floor, forming a straight line.

3 Smoothly and with control, return to the starting position.

4 Repeat on the other side, working up to 10 repetitions on alternating sides.

BENEFITS
- Strengthens and tones shoulders and legs

PERFORMANCE BOOST
- Tennis
- Swimming
- All field sports

DO IT RIGHT
- Keep your torso facing forward as you lunge to the side.
- Pull your abdominal muscles inward.
- Gaze forward.

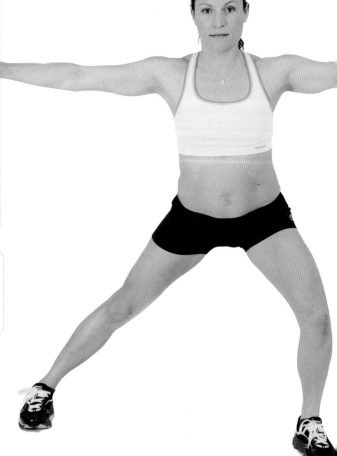

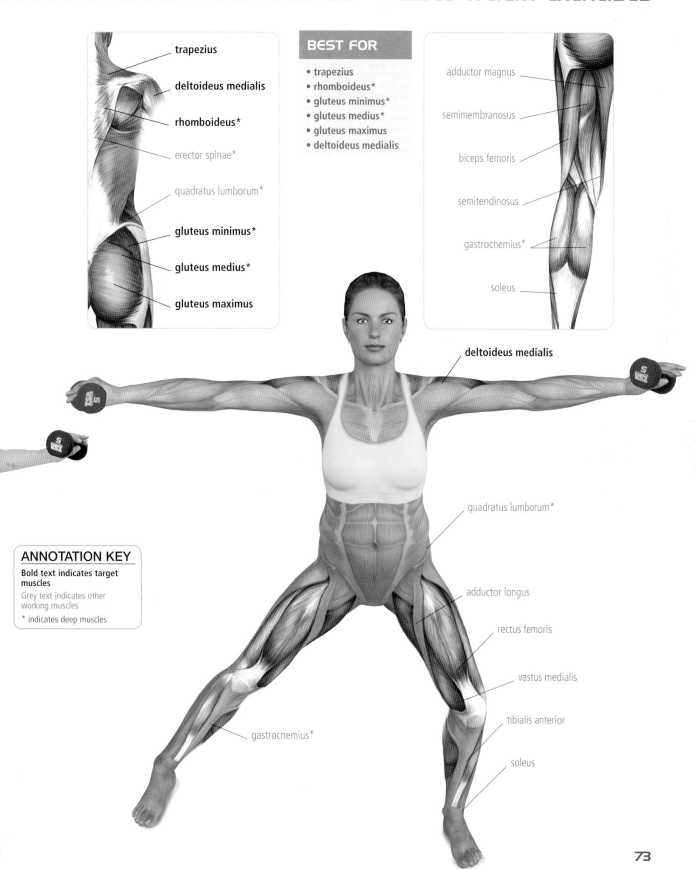

trapezius

deltoideus medialis

rhomboideus*

erector spinae*

quadratus lumborum*

gluteus minimus*

gluteus medius*

gluteus maximus

BEST FOR

- trapezius
- rhomboideus*
- gluteus minimus*
- gluteus medius*
- gluteus maximus
- deltoideus medialis

adductor magnus

semimembranosus

biceps femoris

semitendinosus

gastrocnemius*

soleus

deltoideus medialis

quadratus lumborum*

adductor longus

rectus femoris

vastus medialis

tibialis anterior

soleus

gastrocnemius*

ANNOTATION KEY

Bold text indicates target muscles

Grey text indicates other working muscles

* indicates deep muscles

CURLING STEP-AND-RAISE

❶ Stand with your feet hip-width apart and your arms at your sides, a dumbbell in each hand. Position a step beside your left foot.

❷ Place your left foot on the step.

❸ Shift your weight onto your left foot. Bend your elbows, curling the dumbbells toward your chest. At the same time, raise your right knee as the foot comes off the floor. Continue raising and curling until your right leg forms a right angle and your dumbbells are nearly at shoulder height.

❹ Lowering the dumbbells, cross your right leg over your left leg, which should bend slightly as you lower your right leg to the floor, left of the platform. Simultaneously bend your left leg slightly.

AVOID
- Twisting your neck.
- Hunching your shoulders.
- Arching your back or hunching forward.
- Rushing through the movement.

BENEFITS
- Strengthens and tones abdominal muscles, hips, and biceps
- Improves coordination

PERFORMANCE BOOST
- All field sports
- Stair-climbing

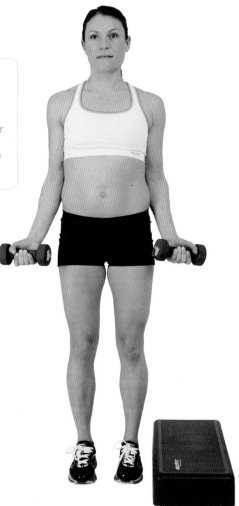

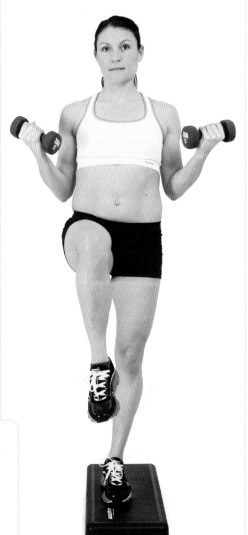

DO IT RIGHT
- Keep your upper arms stationary as you curl and release.
- Keep your movements smooth and controlled.
- Keep your torso facing forward.
- Pull your abdominal muscles inward.
- Gaze forward.
- Press your shoulders away from your ears.

BEST FOR

- adductor magnus
- rectus abdominis
- tensor fasciae latae
- adductor longus
- biceps brachii

ANNOTATION KEY

Bold text indicates target muscles

Grey text indicates other working muscles

* indicates deep muscles

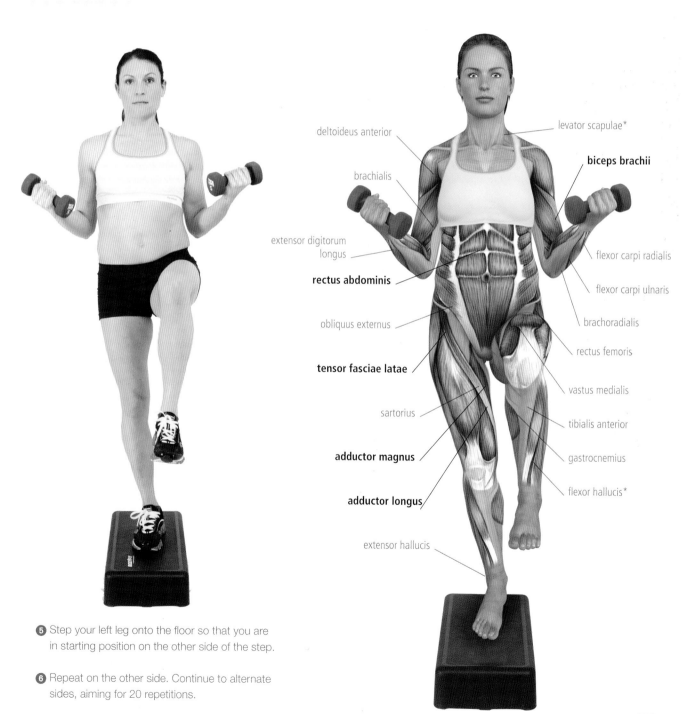

deltoideus anterior

brachialis

extensor digitorum longus

rectus abdominis

obliquus externus

tensor fasciae latae

sartorius

adductor magnus

adductor longus

extensor hallucis

levator scapulae*

biceps brachii

flexor carpi radialis

flexor carpi ulnaris

brachoradialis

rectus femoris

vastus medialis

tibialis anterior

gastrocnemius

flexor hallucis*

5 Step your left leg onto the floor so that you are in starting position on the other side of the step.

6 Repeat on the other side. Continue to alternate sides, aiming for 20 repetitions.

FIGURE 8

1 Stand with your feet hip-width apart or slightly wider. Grasp a medicine ball in both hands, and hold it in front of your torso.

2 Shift your weight to the right. In a smooth, controlled movement, extend both arms and bring the medicine ball toward the lower right side of your body.

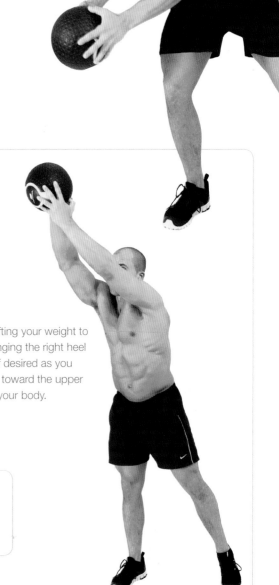

AVOID
- Straining your neck.
- Tensing or hunching your shoulders.
- Arching your back or hunching forward.
- Rushing through the movement.

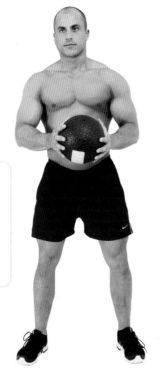

BENEFITS
- Improves coordination, flexibility and range of motion
- Strengthens and tones core and arm muscles
- Stabilises core

PERFORMANCE BOOST
- Tennis
- Squash
- Basketball
- Baseball
- Swimming

3 Continue shifting your weight to the right, bringing the right heel off the floor if desired as you raise the ball toward the upper right side of your body.

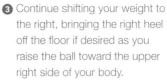

DO IT RIGHT
- Follow the ball's movement with your gaze.
- Keep your core muscles engaged and your abs pulled inward.
- Anchor both feet to the floor.

FIGURE 8 • ADDED-WEIGHT EXERCISES

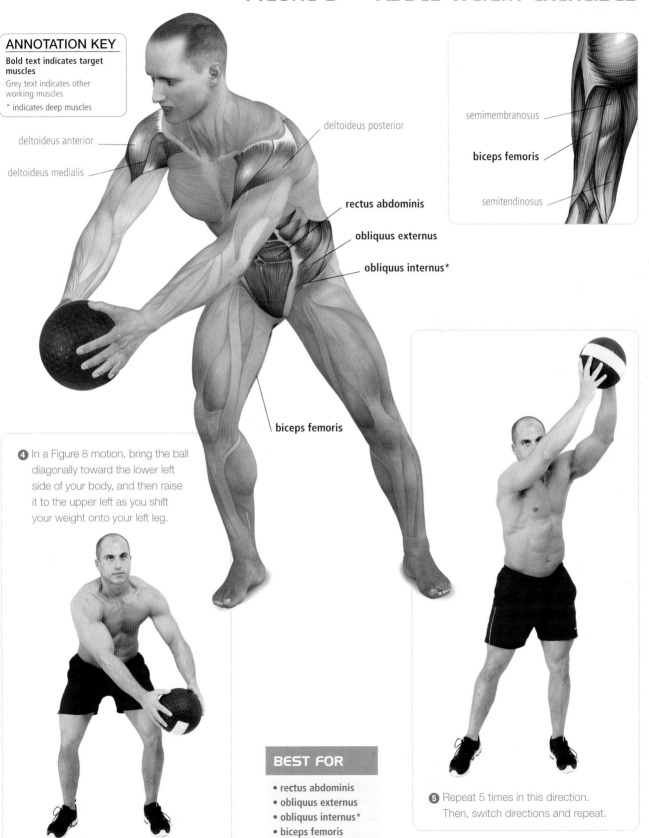

ANNOTATION KEY

Bold text indicates target muscles

Grey text indicates other working muscles

* indicates deep muscles

deltoideus anterior

deltoideus medialis

deltoideus posterior

rectus abdominis

obliquus externus

obliquus internus*

biceps femoris

semimembranosus

biceps femoris

semitendinosus

❹ In a Figure 8 motion, bring the ball diagonally toward the lower left side of your body, and then raise it to the upper left as you shift your weight onto your left leg.

BEST FOR

• rectus abdominis
• obliquus externus
• obliquus internus*
• biceps femoris

❺ Repeat 5 times in this direction. Then, switch directions and repeat.

KNEE RAISE WITH LATERAL EXTENSION

❶ Stand with your feet hip-width apart and your arms at your sides, a dumbbell in each hand.

❷ Shifting weight onto your left leg, bend your right knee and raise the leg. At the same time, raise your arms until the weights are slightly below shoulder height. Take a moment or two to find your balance.

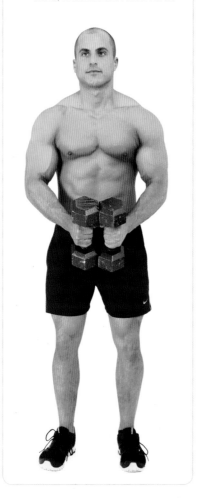

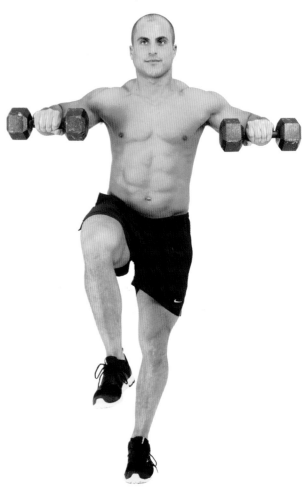

BENEFITS
- Improves balance, coordination, and range of motion
- Strengthens and tones core, shoulder, chest and arm muscles
- Stabilses core

PERFORMANCE BOOST
- Football
- Tennis
- Squash
- Baseball
- Rollerblading and skating
- Skiing

AVOID
- Twisting your torso to either side.
- Letting your abs bulge outward.
- Arching your back or hunching forward.

DO IT RIGHT
- Keep your torso facing forward as much as possible.
- Pull your navel toward your spine and engage your abdominal muscles.
- Gaze forward.
- Maintain a neutral S-curve in your spine.
- Anchor your standing leg to the floor.
- Keep breathing.

❸ Keeping your arms and upper body stationary, extend your right leg out to the side. Try holding for a few seconds.

❹ Moving with control, lower your arms and return your right leg to starting position.

❺ Repeat on the other side. Alternating sides, begin with 5 repetitions on each side before working up to 10.

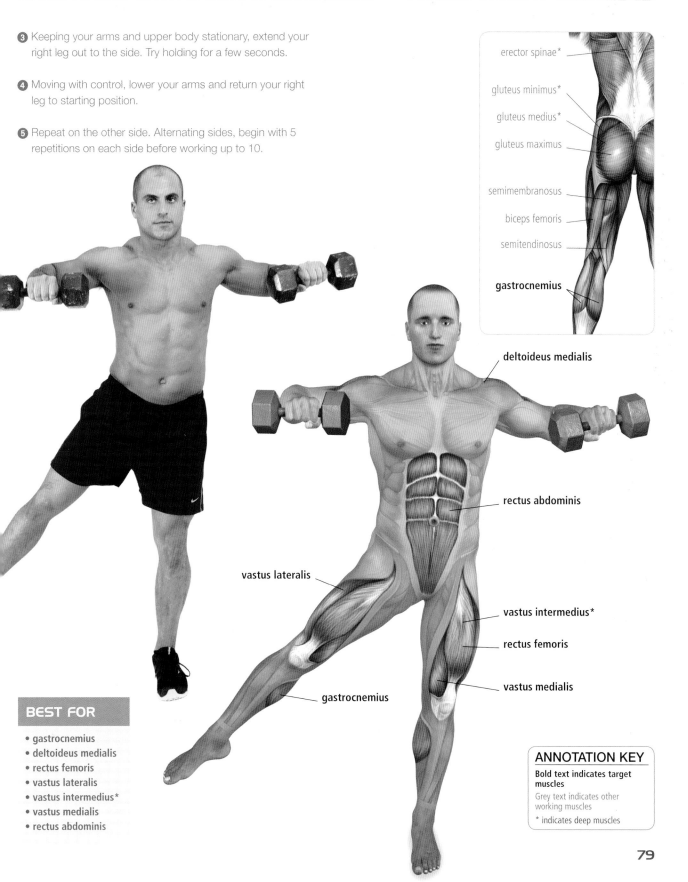

erector spinae*

gluteus minimus*

gluteus medius*

gluteus maximus

semimembranosus

biceps femoris

semitendinosus

gastrocnemius

deltoideus medialis

rectus abdominis

vastus lateralis

vastus intermedius*

rectus femoris

vastus medialis

gastrocnemius

BEST FOR

- gastrocnemius
- deltoideus medialis
- rectus femoris
- vastus lateralis
- vastus intermedius*
- vastus medialis
- rectus abdominis

ANNOTATION KEY

Bold text indicates target muscles

Grey text indicates other working muscles

* indicates deep muscles

79

DEAD LIFT

1 Stand with your feet shoulder-width apart, with a barbell at your feet. Lean over to grasp the weight with both hands.

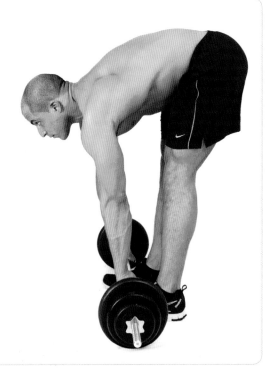

2 Using your core muscles as well as your arms, raise the barbell, hingeing at the hips as you slowly rise to a standing position.

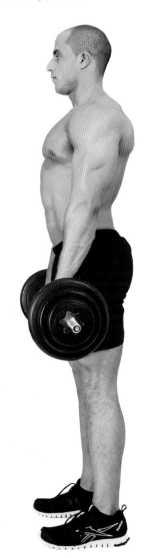

BENEFITS
• Strengthens and tones core and arm muscles

PERFORMANCE BOOST
• Tennis
• Squash
• Baseball

DO IT RIGHT
• Maintain a slight bend in your knees if desired.
• As much as possible, maintain a neutral S-shaped spinal position as you lift and lower.
• Spend just as much time lowering as you spend lifting.
• Engage your chest and shoulders.
• Gaze forward.

AVOID
• Feeling a sense of collapse in your chest and shoulders.
• Hunching your shoulders.
• Moving in a jerky manner.
• Taking on too much weight at once.
• Arching your back or excessively hunching it forward.
• Performing this exercise if you experience lower-back pain.

BEST FOR

- erector spinae*
- gluteus maximus
- adductor magnus
- biceps femoris
- semitendinosus
- semimembranosus

ANNOTATION KEY

Bold text indicates target muscles

Grey text indicates other working muscles

* indicates deep muscles

3 Smoothly return the barbell to the floor, again hingeing at the hips. Repeat, starting with 3 repetitions before building up to 10.

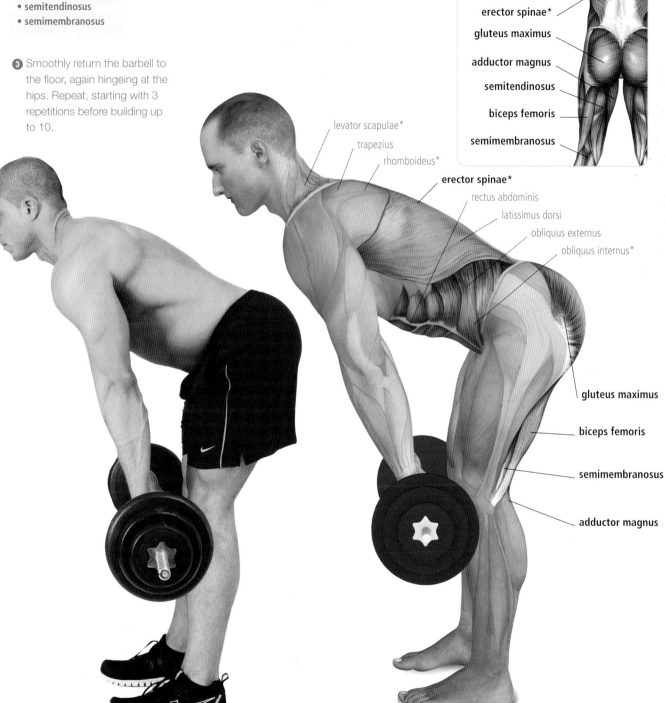

levator scapulae*

trapezius

rhomboideus*

latissimus dorsi

erector spinae*

gluteus maximus

adductor magnus

semitendinosus

biceps femoris

semimembranosus

levator scapulae*

trapezius

rhomboideus*

erector spinae*

rectus abdominis

latissimus dorsi

obliquus externus

obliquus internus*

gluteus maximus

biceps femoris

semimembranosus

adductor magnus

ROLL-UP TRICEPS LIFT

❶ Lie on the floor, with your spine in a neutral position. Hold a body bar in both hands. Bend your elbows so that your arms form a right angle with the body bar above your head.

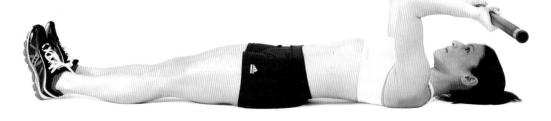

AVOID
- Moving in a jerky manner.
- Twisting your torso or moving your hips off the floor.

❷ Keeping the rest of your body in place, straighten your arms.

BENEFITS
- Strengthens and tones core muscles and triceps

PERFORMANCE BOOST
- Dance
- Gymnastics

❸ Maintaining this arm position, use your core muscles to smoothly roll up to a sitting position. Keep your arms extended, with the body bar lifted overhead.

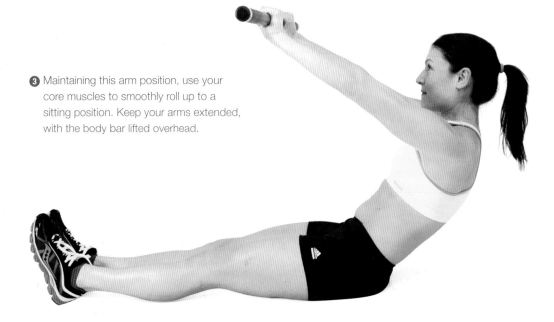

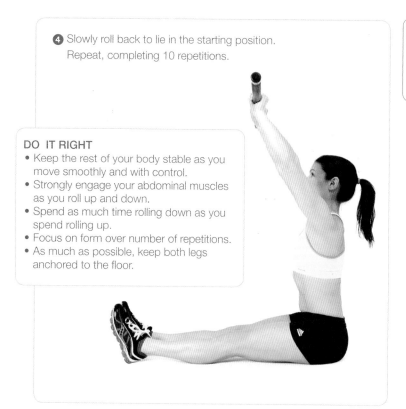

④ Slowly roll back to lie in the starting position. Repeat, completing 10 repetitions.

DO IT RIGHT

- Keep the rest of your body stable as you move smoothly and with control.
- Strongly engage your abdominal muscles as you roll up and down.
- Spend as much time rolling down as you spend rolling up.
- Focus on form over number of repetitions.
- As much as possible, keep both legs anchored to the floor.

ANNOTATION KEY

Bold text indicates target muscles

Grey text indicates other working muscles

* indicates deep muscles

BEST FOR

- erector spinae*
- triceps brachii
- obliquus externus
- rectus abdominis
- transversus abdominis*

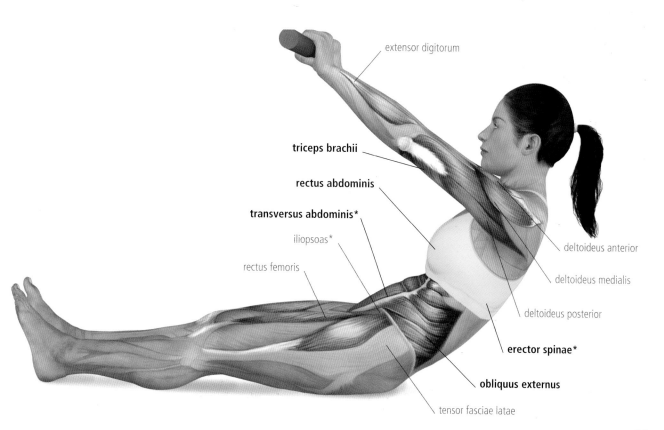

extensor digitorum

triceps brachii

rectus abdominis

transversus abdominis*

iliopsoas*

rectus femoris

deltoideus anterior

deltoideus medialis

deltoideus posterior

erector spinae*

obliquus externus

tensor fasciae latae

LYING ABDUCTION

❶ Lie on your side, with one leg stacked on top of the other and one arm supporting you, forearm on the floor and palm down. Extend the other arm along the side of your body, a dumbbell in your hand.

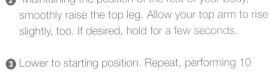

DO IT RIGHT
- Lower your leg just as smoothly as you lift it.
- Keep your torso facing forward.
- Keep your legs extended.
- Anchor your bottom arm and leg to the floor.
- Gaze forward.

AVOID
- Tilting or twisting your hips as you raise your leg.
- Tensing or twisting your neck.
- Hunching your shoulders.

BENEFITS
- Strengthens and tones outer legs and core

PERFORMANCE BOOST
- Tennis
- All field sports

❷ Maintaining the position of the rest of your body, smoothly raise the top leg. Allow your top arm to rise slightly, too. If desired, hold for a few seconds.

❸ Lower to starting position. Repeat, performing 10 repetitions before switching sides and repeating.

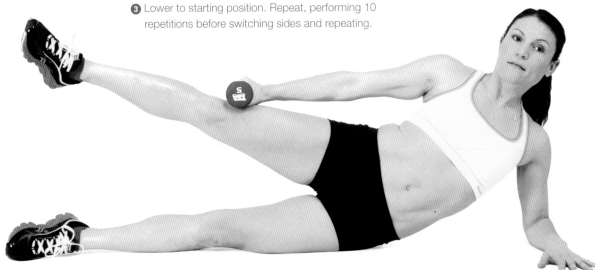

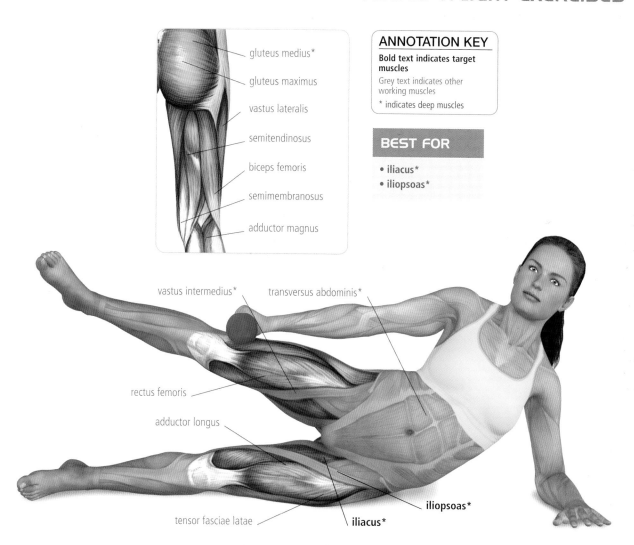

gluteus medius*
gluteus maximus
vastus lateralis
semitendinosus
biceps femoris
semimembranosus
adductor magnus

ANNOTATION KEY

Bold text indicates target muscles

Grey text indicates other working muscles

* indicates deep muscles

BEST FOR

- **iliacus***
- **iliopsoas***

vastus intermedius*
transversus abdominis*
rectus femoris
adductor longus
iliopsoas*
tensor fasciae latae
iliacus*

MODIFICATION

Harder: Try moving into a side plank position. Focus on keeping your body in a straight line as you hold.

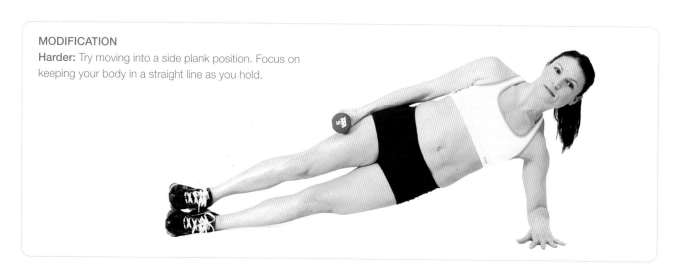

SEATED RUSSIAN TWIST

1 Holding a dumbbell in both hands, sit with your legs extended in front of you, knees bent and feet about hip-width apart. Lean back slightly.

DO IT RIGHT
- Engage your core.
- Anchor your heels to the floor.
- Move smoothly.

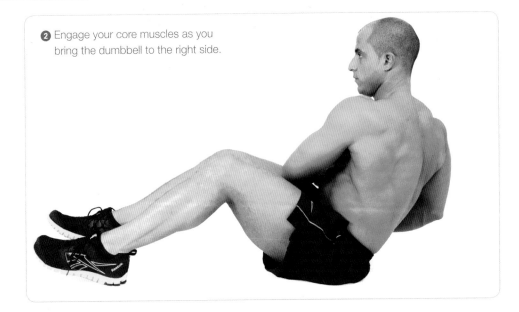

2 Engage your core muscles as you bring the dumbbell to the right side.

BENEFITS
- Strengthens core, especially obliques, lower-back extensors, abdominals and deep core stabilisers

PERFORMANCE BOOST
- Tennis
- Baseball
- Bowling

AVOID
- Arching or rounding your back.
- Hunching your shoulders.
- Swinging your arms or moving in a jerky manner.
- Allowing your heels to lift off the floor.
- Tensing your neck as you twist.

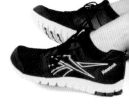

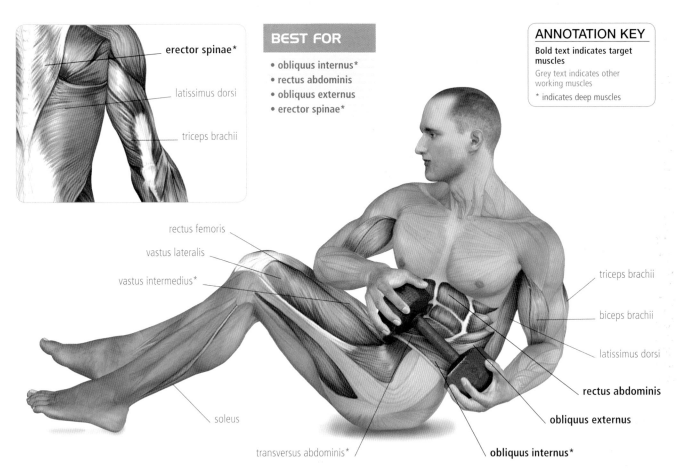

erector spinae*

latissimus dorsi

triceps brachii

BEST FOR

• obliquus internus*
• rectus abdominis
• obliquus externus
• erector spinae*

ANNOTATION KEY

Bold text indicates target muscles

Grey text indicates other working muscles

* indicates deep muscles

rectus femoris

vastus lateralis

vastus intermedius*

soleus

transversus abdominis*

triceps brachii

biceps brachii

latissimus dorsi

rectus abdominis

obliquus externus

obliquus internus*

❸ Bring the dumbbell to the middle of your body and then to the left side. Repeat, performing 20 rotations.

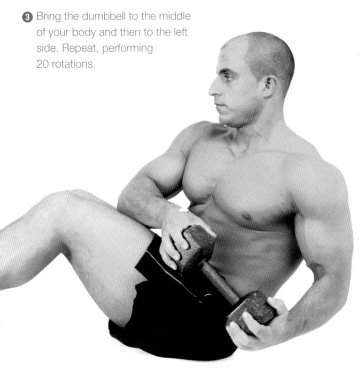

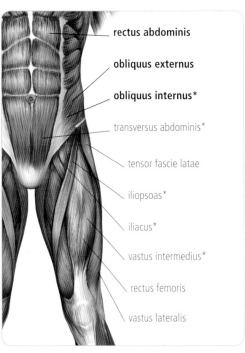

rectus abdominis

obliquus externus

obliquus internus*

transversus abdominis*

tensor fascie latae

iliopsoas*

iliacus*

vastus intermedius*

rectus femoris

vastus lateralis

SWISS BALL PULLOVER

❶ Lie face-up on the Swiss ball, with your upper back and neck supported. Your body should be extended with your torso long, legs bent with knees directly over ankles, and feet planted on the floor slightly wider than shoulder-distance apart. Using both hands, grasp a dumbbell and extend your arms behind you, level with your shoulders so that your body from knees to fingertips forms a long line.

AVOID
- Locking your arms when they are extended behind your head.
- Arching your back.
- Rushing through the exercise.
- Rolling excessively on the ball.

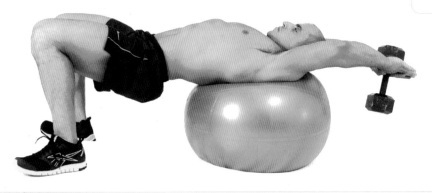

BENEFITS
- Stabilises core muscles
- Strengthens upper back

PERFORMANCE BOOST
- Tennis
- Basketball
- Baseball

❷ Keeping the rest of your body stable and your arms as straight as possible, raise your arms upward.

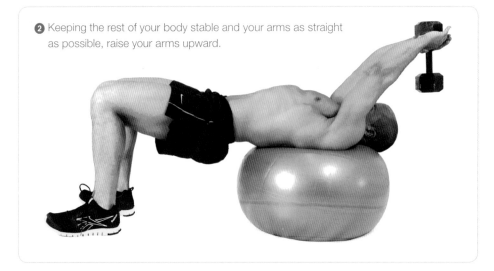

DO IT RIGHT
- Keep your torso stable.
- Anchor both feet to the floor.
- Engage your abdominal muscles.
- Keep your buttocks and pelvis lifted so that your upper legs, torso and neck form a line.
- Lower your arms just as smoothly as you raise them.

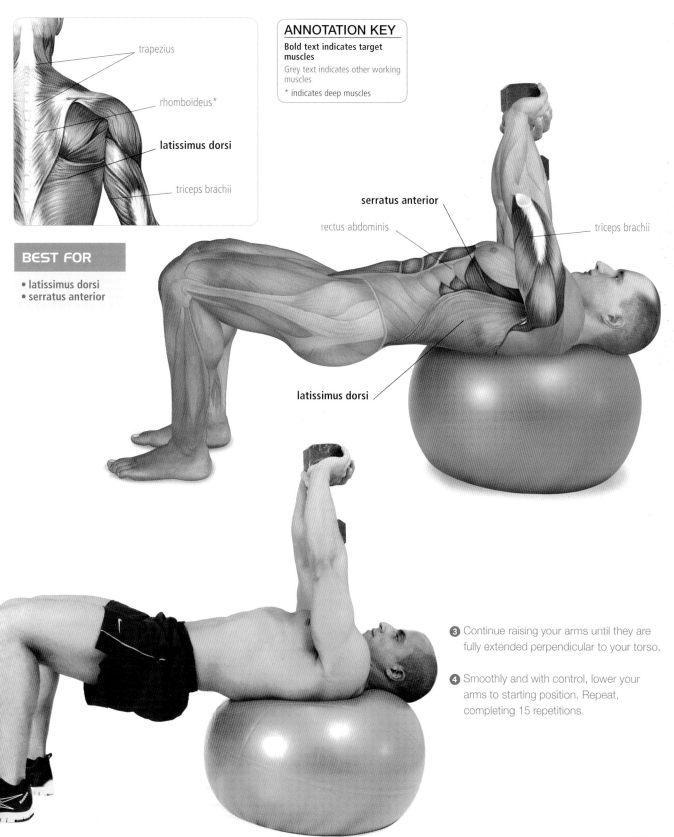

trapezius

rhomboideus*

latissimus dorsi

triceps brachii

ANNOTATION KEY
Bold text indicates target muscles
Grey text indicates other working muscles
* indicates deep muscles

serratus anterior

rectus abdominis

triceps brachii

latissimus dorsi

BEST FOR
• latissimus dorsi
• serratus anterior

❸ Continue raising your arms until they are fully extended perpendicular to your torso.

❹ Smoothly and with control, lower your arms to starting position. Repeat, completing 15 repetitions.

BALL SQUAT WITH BICEPS CURL

1 Stand at a wall, with the Swiss ball against your back, grasping a dumbbell in each hand. Plant your feet slightly in front of your torso to prepare.

DO IT RIGHT
- Engage your core muscles; your abs should be driving the movement.
- Keep your hips facing forward.
- Gaze forward.
- Maintain the line of your torso as you squat and rise to stand.

AVOID
- Rushing through the movement.
- Losing control of the ball.
- Twisting your hips to either side.

BENEFITS
- Strengthens and tones legs, biceps, core and gluteal muscles

PERFORMANCE BOOST
- Dance
- Gymnastics
- All sports requiring balance

2 Bend your knees and lower toward the floor while curling the dumbbells toward your chest. As you lower into the squat position, keep the Swiss ball behind your back.

3 Gradually straighten your arms and legs as you rise to stand and release the dumbbells to your sides. Repeat, carrying out 15 repetitions.

MODIFICATION

Harder: While in the squatting and curling position, extend one leg, hold and release. Repeat on the other side.

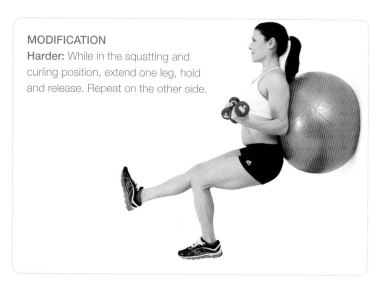

BEST FOR

- **brachialis**
- **brachioradialis**
- **biceps brachii**
- **rectus femoris**
- **vastus lateralis**
- **vastus intermedius***
- **vastus medialis**
- **gluteus maximus**
- **biceps femoris**
- **semitendinosus**
- **semimembranosus**

ANNOTATION KEY

Bold text indicates target muscles

Grey text indicates other working muscles

* indicates deep muscles

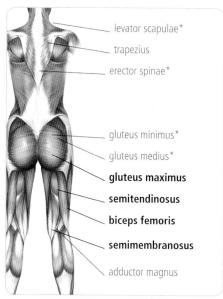

levator scapulae*
trapezius
erector spinae*
gluteus minimus*
gluteus medius*
gluteus maximus
semitendinosus
biceps femoris
semimembranosus
adductor magnus

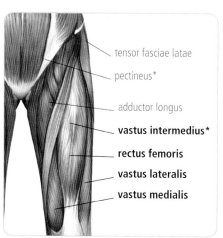

tensor fasciae latae
pectineus*
adductor longus
vastus intermedius*
rectus femoris
vastus lateralis
vastus medialis

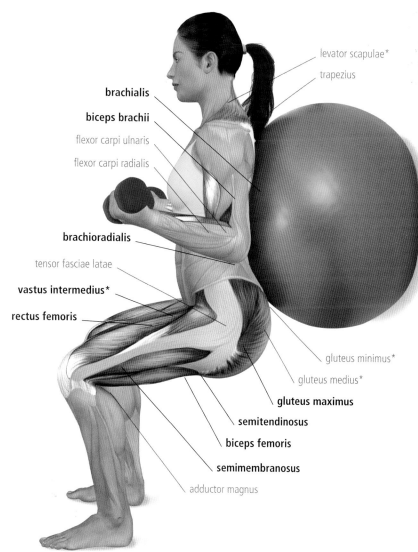

brachialis
biceps brachii
flexor carpi ulnaris
flexor carpi radialis
brachioradialis
tensor fasciae latae
vastus intermedius*
rectus femoris

levator scapulae*
trapezius
gluteus minimus*
gluteus medius*
gluteus maximus
semitendinosus
biceps femoris
semimembranosus
adductor magnus

LATERAL STEP AND CURL

① Stand with your feet hip-width apart and your arms at your sides, a dumbbell in each hand. Position a step beside your right foot.

② Step to the right, placing your right foot on the step. Simultaneously bend your elbows, curling the dumbbells into your chest.

③ Lowering the dumbbells, bring your left leg onto the step.

④ Curl the dumbbells into your chest as you step your right leg off of the step. Release the dumbbells as you step down with your left leg. You should now be in the starting position with the step to your right.

AVOID
- Twisting your neck.
- Hunching your shoulders.
- Arching your back or hunching forward.
- Moving so quickly that you sacrifice form.

BENEFITS
- Strengthens and tones legs and arms

PERFORMANCE BOOST
- Tennis
- Squash
- All field sports, especially football

DO IT RIGHT
- Keep your upper arms stationary as you curl and release.
- Keep your movements smooth and controlled.
- Keep your torso facing forward.
- Pull your abdominal muscles inward.
- Gaze forward.
- Press your shoulders away from your ears.

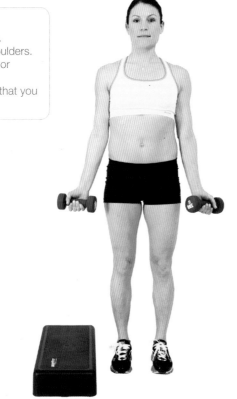

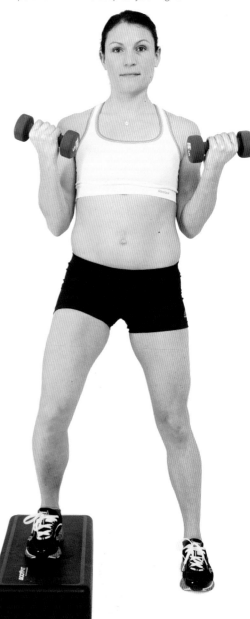

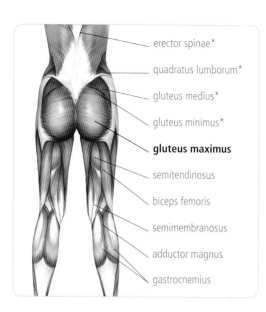

- erector spinae*
- quadratus lumborum*
- gluteus medius*
- gluteus minimus*
- **gluteus maximus**
- semitendinosus
- biceps femoris
- semimembranosus
- adductor magnus
- gastrocnemius

ANNOTATION KEY

Bold text indicates target muscles

Grey text indicates other working muscles

* indicates deep muscles

BEST FOR

- **biceps brachii**
- **vastus intermedius***
- **rectus femoris***
- **vastus lateralis**
- **vastus medialis**
- **gluteus maximus**

5 Repeat, stepping to the left this time. Keeping a steady pace, complete 20 repetitions.

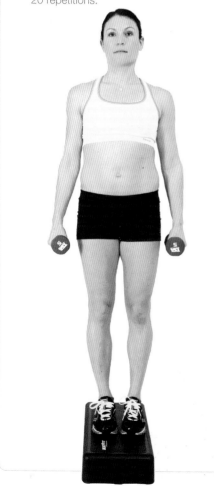

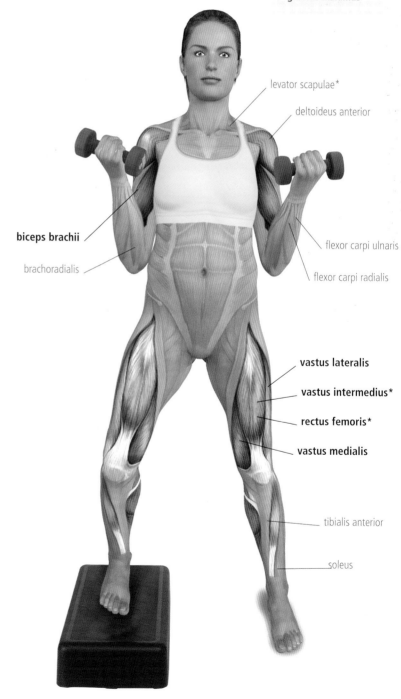

- levator scapulae*
- deltoideus anterior
- **biceps brachii**
- brachoradialis
- flexor carpi ulnaris
- flexor carpi radialis
- **vastus lateralis**
- **vastus intermedius***
- **rectus femoris***
- **vastus medialis**
- tibialis anterior
- soleus

CROSSOVER STEP-UP

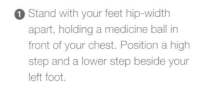

❶ Stand with your feet hip-width apart, holding a medicine ball in front of your chest. Position a high step and a lower step beside your left foot.

❷ Cross your right leg over your left, resting it on the step. Shift weight onto this right foot to step up.

BENEFITS
- Improves agility and coordination
- Stabilises core

PERFORMANCE BOOST
- Tennis
- Squash
- Football
- Rugby
- Rollerblading and skating

AVOID
- Twisting your neck.
- Hunching your shoulders.
- Arching your back or hunching forward.
- Moving so quickly that you sacrifice form.

❸ Rest your left foot on the lower step.

❹ Again cross your right leg over your left to step down onto the floor.

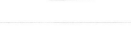

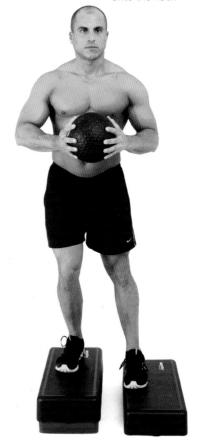

DO IT RIGHT
- Keep holding the medicine ball in front of your chest.
- Maintain a steady pace.
- Keep your torso facing forward.
- Pull your abdominal muscles inward.
- Gaze forward.
- Press your shoulders away from your ears.

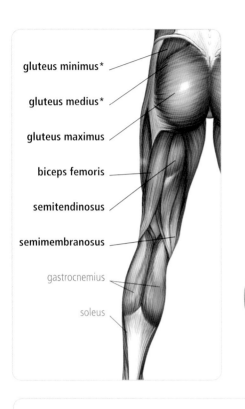

gluteus minimus*

gluteus medius*

gluteus maximus

biceps femoris

semitendinosus

semimembranosus

gastrocnemius

soleus

BEST FOR

- rectus femoris
- vastus lateralis
- vastus intermedius*
- vastus medialis
- biceps femoris
- semitendinosus
- semimembranosus
- gluteus maximus
- gluteus medius*
- gluteus minimus*

ANNOTATION KEY

Bold text indicates target muscles

Grey text indicates other working muscles

* indicates deep muscles

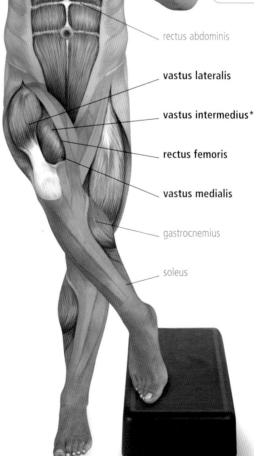

rectus abdominis

vastus lateralis

vastus intermedius*

rectus femoris

vastus medialis

gastrocnemius

soleus

5 Step your right leg onto the floor so that you are standing to the left of the step.

6 Repeat in the other direction. Perform 15 repetitions.

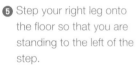

OBSTACLE CHALLENGE

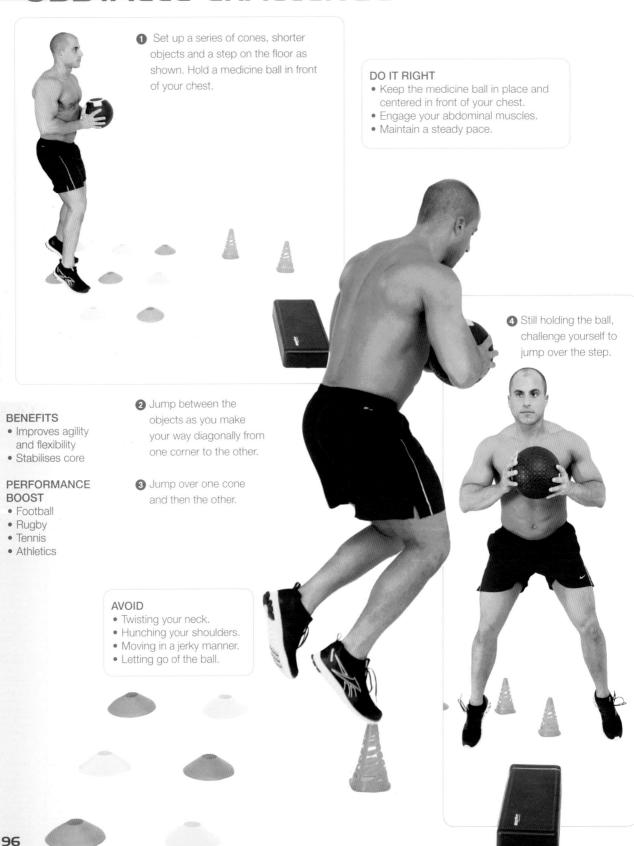

1 Set up a series of cones, shorter objects and a step on the floor as shown. Hold a medicine ball in front of your chest.

DO IT RIGHT
- Keep the medicine ball in place and centered in front of your chest.
- Engage your abdominal muscles.
- Maintain a steady pace.

4 Still holding the ball, challenge yourself to jump over the step.

BENEFITS
- Improves agility and flexibility
- Stabilises core

PERFORMANCE BOOST
- Football
- Rugby
- Tennis
- Athletics

2 Jump between the objects as you make your way diagonally from one corner to the other.

3 Jump over one cone and then the other.

AVOID
- Twisting your neck.
- Hunching your shoulders.
- Moving in a jerky manner.
- Letting go of the ball.

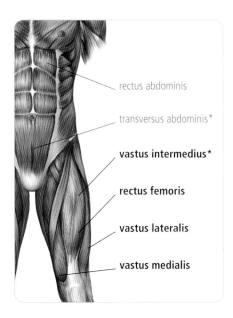

rectus abdominis

transversus abdominis*

vastus intermedius*

rectus femoris

vastus lateralis

vastus medialis

ANNOTATION KEY

Bold text indicates target muscles

Grey text indicates other working muscles

* indicates deep muscles

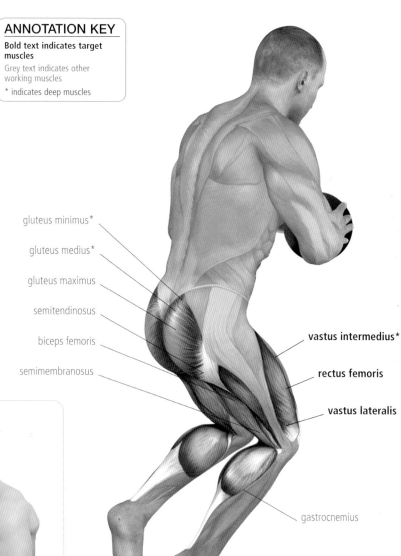

gluteus minimus*

gluteus medius*

gluteus maximus

semitendinosus

biceps femoris

semimembranosus

vastus intermedius*

rectus femoris

vastus lateralis

gastrocnemius

5 Jog back from the step to the beginning of the course. Begin again, completing the course up to 10 times.

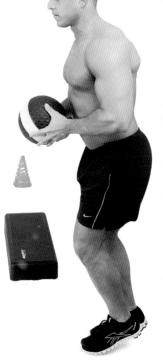

BEST FOR

- rectus femoris
- vastus lateralis
- vastus intermedius*
- vastus medialis

97

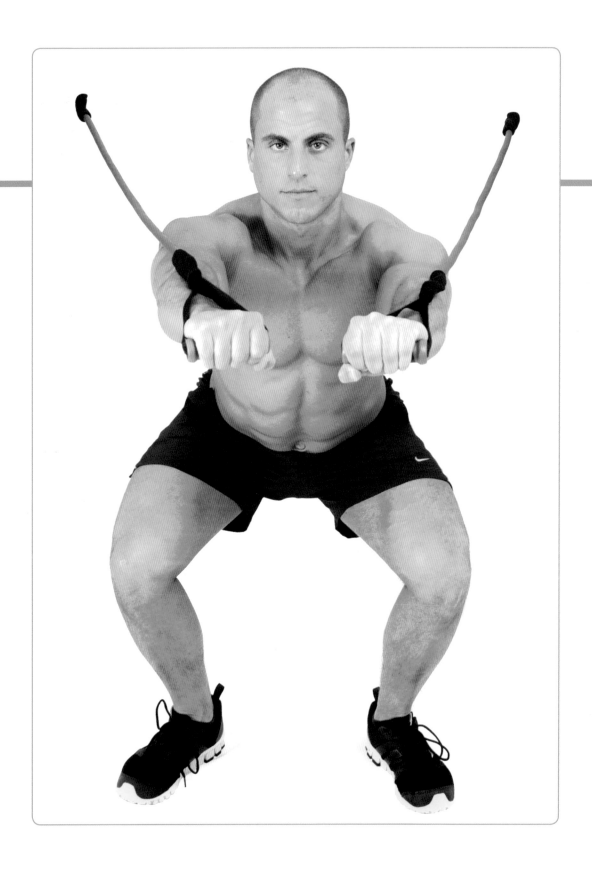

RESISTANCE EXERCISES

The following resistance exercises are designed to build power within your body. Feel free to experiment with the equipment; for instance, swap dumbbells for a medicine ball or increase the weight on your machine. Whether exercising in the gym or at home, avoid moving in a jerky manner; instead, perform these exercises smoothly, deliberately, and with control, maintaining your form and breathing continuously. For motivation, study each exercise's muscle diagram and picture yourself growing stronger, leaner and more toned with every single repetition.

WOODCHOP

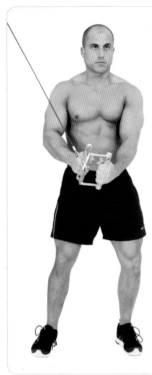

1 Stand with your feet slightly wider than hip-distance part, with each weight machine to your right. Grasp the handle of the cable in both hands. Your legs may be slightly bent.

AVOID
- Locking your knees.
- Hunching your shoulders.
- Twisting your neck.
- Moving in a jerky manner from side to side.
- Raising your arms so high that you lose control of your core and/or arch your back.

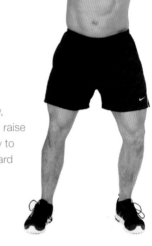

2 Slowly and smoothly, rotate your core and raise your arms diagonally to the upper right, toward the cable machine.

BENEFITS
- Strengthens and tones arms and oblique muscles
- Builds endurance

PERFORMANCE BOOST
- Golf
- Tennis
- Skiing

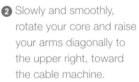
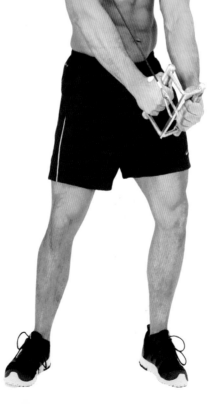

DO IT RIGHT
- Move slowly and with control.
- Follow your arms with your gaze as you raise and lower.
- Keep your core contracted and your abs engaged.
- You can also perform this exercise with a resistance band, anchoring one end beneath one foot, holding the other end in both hands, and twisting in the opposite direction.

3 In a controlled 'chopping' motion, bring your arms diagonally back to starting position and then down to the other side, rotating your core away from the machine.

4 Complete 10 repetitions. Then, switch sides and repeat.

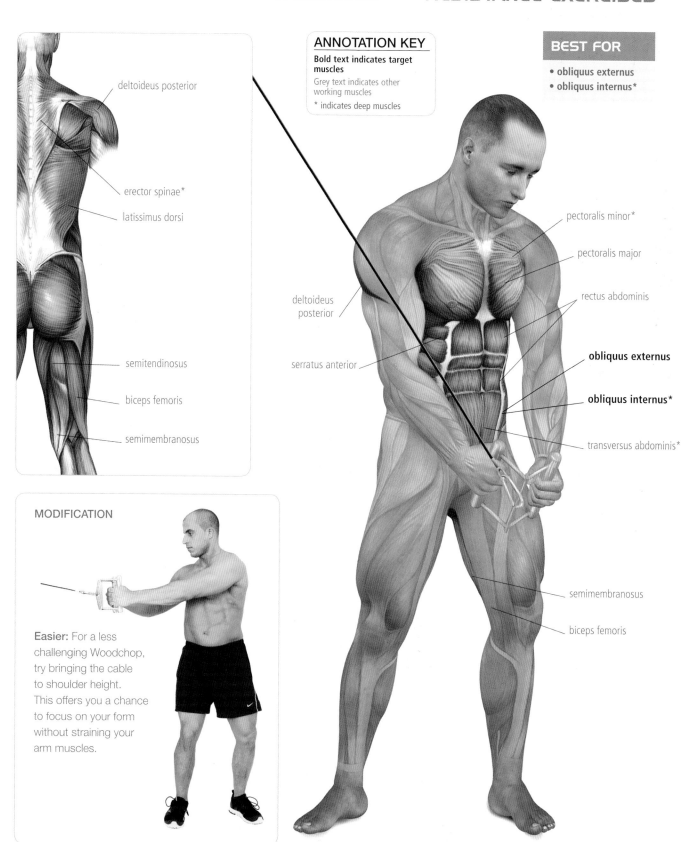

ANNOTATION KEY

Bold text indicates target muscles

Grey text indicates other working muscles

* indicates deep muscles

BEST FOR

- **obliquus externus**
- **obliquus internus***

deltoideus posterior

erector spinae*

latissimus dorsi

semitendinosus

biceps femoris

semimembranosus

pectoralis minor*

pectoralis major

rectus abdominis

obliquus externus

obliquus internus*

transversus abdominis*

deltoideus posterior

serratus anterior

semimembranosus

biceps femoris

MODIFICATION

Easier: For a less challenging Woodchop, try bringing the cable to shoulder height. This offers you a chance to focus on your form without straining your arm muscles.

TWISTING LIFT

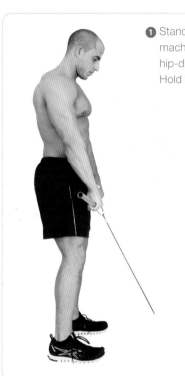

1 Stand upright, facing a cable machine, with your feet planted hip-distance apart or slightly wider. Hold the cable in both hands.

DO IT RIGHT
- Keep your feet planted and your torso stable as you move.
- Move slowly and with control.
- Keep your abdominal and gluteal muscles engaged throughout.

BENEFITS
- Strengthens and tones arms and oblique muscles
- Builds endurance

PERFORMANCE BOOST
- Golf
- Tennis
- Skiing

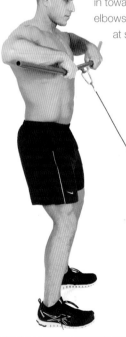

2 In a smooth movement, pull the cable toward your body as you bend your elbows to bring the cable in toward your chest. Your elbows should be almost at shoulder height.

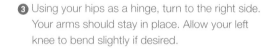

3 Using your hips as a hinge, turn to the right side. Your arms should stay in place. Allow your left knee to bend slightly if desired.

3 Gradually twist back to starting position, facing the machine.

4 Straighten your arms, releasing the cable to return to starting position. Switch sides and repeat, aiming for 20 per side.

AVOID
- Moving in a jerky manner.
- Locking your knees.
- Arching your back or slumping forward.

BEST FOR

- trapezius
- deltoideus medialis
- rectus abdominis
- obliquus externus
- obliquus internus*

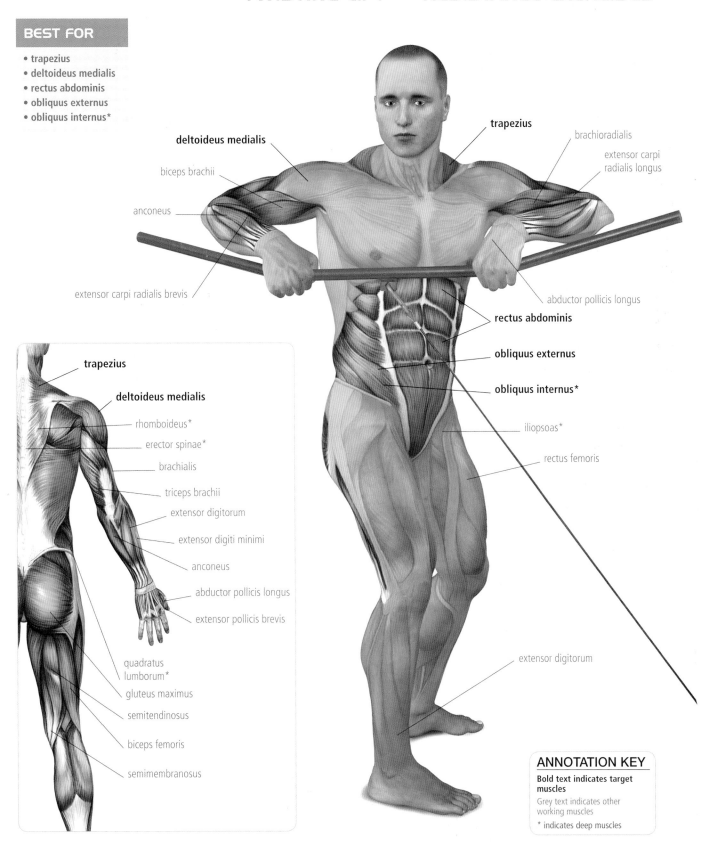

deltoideus medialis

biceps brachii

anconeus

extensor carpi radialis brevis

trapezius

brachioradialis

extensor carpi radialis longus

abductor pollicis longus

rectus abdominis

obliquus externus

obliquus internus*

iliopsoas*

rectus femoris

extensor digitorum

trapezius

deltoideus medialis

rhomboideus*

erector spinae*

brachialis

triceps brachii

extensor digitorum

extensor digiti minimi

anconeus

abductor pollicis longus

extensor pollicis brevis

quadratus lumborum*

gluteus maximus

semitendinosus

biceps femoris

semimembranosus

ANNOTATION KEY

Bold text indicates target muscles

Grey text indicates other working muscles

* indicates deep muscles

SQUAT AND ROW

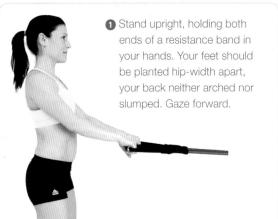

1 Stand upright, holding both ends of a resistance band in your hands. Your feet should be planted hip-width apart, your back neither arched nor slumped. Gaze forward.

2 In a smooth movement, begin to bend your knees. At the same time, bend your elbows as you pull both ends of the band in toward your body.

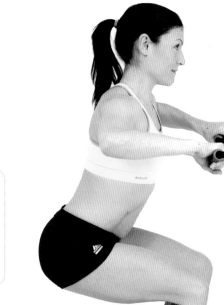

DO IT RIGHT
- Keep both feet anchored to the ground.
- When bending, aim for your legs to form a right angle.
- Move slowly and with control.
- Keep your belly pulled inward.

BENEFITS
- Strengthens and tones leg, gluteal and shoulder muscles
- Builds endurance

PERFORMANCE BOOST
- Skiing
- Skating and rollerblading
- Rowing

3 Keeping the rest of your body stable and your abdominal muscles engaged, use both hands to pull the band even further toward your body.

4 Smoothly return to starting position. Repeat, starting with 10 repetitions and building up to 20.

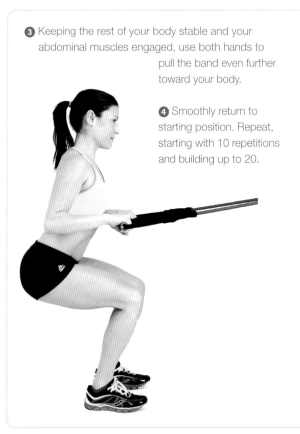

AVOID
- Twisting your torso.
- Arching your back.
- Rushing through the movement.
- Twisting your neck to either side.
- Lowering your chin.

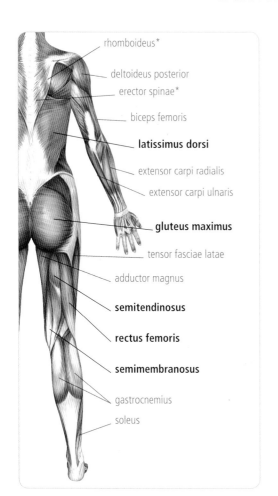

rhomboideus*
deltoideus posterior
erector spinae*
biceps femoris
latissimus dorsi
extensor carpi radialis
extensor carpi ulnaris
gluteus maximus
tensor fasciae latae
adductor magnus
semitendinosus
rectus femoris
semimembranosus
gastrocnemius
soleus

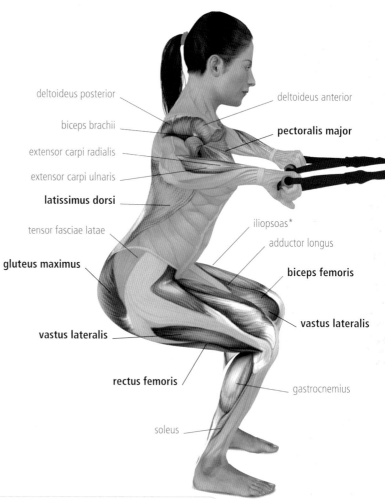

deltoideus posterior
biceps brachii
extensor carpi radialis
extensor carpi ulnaris
latissimus dorsi
tensor fasciae latae
gluteus maximus
vastus lateralis
rectus femoris
soleus

deltoideus anterior
pectoralis major
iliopsoas*
adductor longus
biceps femoris
vastus lateralis
gastrocnemius

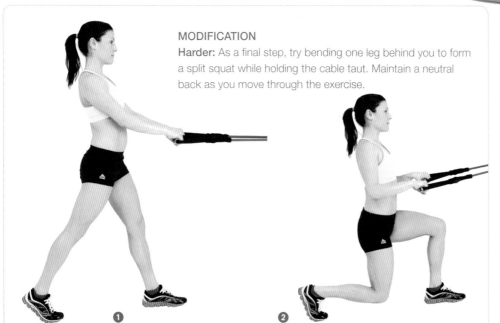

MODIFICATION

Harder: As a final step, try bending one leg behind you to form a split squat while holding the cable taut. Maintain a neutral back as you move through the exercise.

1

2

BEST FOR

- gluteus maximus
- rectus femoris
- vastus lateralis
- vastus intermedius*
- vastus medialis
- biceps femoris
- semitendinosus
- semimembranosus
- latissimus dorsi
- pectoralis major

ANNOTATION KEY

Bold text indicates target muscles

Grey text indicates other working muscles

* indicates deep muscles

REVERSE LUNGE WITH CHEST PRESS

1 Stand upright with your feet roughly hip-width apart. Grasp the handle of one resistance band in each hand. Loop the other handles of both bands around weight machines or other stable objects to either side of you. Raise your arms to hold both bands perpendicular to your body, slightly taut.

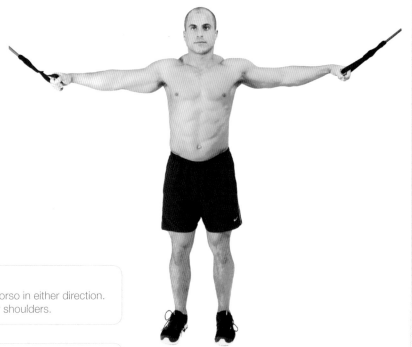

AVOID
- Twisting your torso in either direction.
- Hunching your shoulders.

DO IT RIGHT
- Keep your torso facing forward.
- Engage your abdominal and gluteal muscles.
- Move slowly and with control.

BENEFITS
- Strengthens and tones arms and chest muscles
- Improves coordination

PERFORMANCE BOOST
- Tennis
- Skiing
- All field sports

2 Step your left leg behind you.

3 Bend both knees into a reverse lunge position. At the same time lower both arms, feeling resistance on the bands.

4 Gradually straighten your legs, and raise your arms to your sides to return to starting position.

5 Step your left leg forward, and repeat on the other side. Alternating, aim for 10 repetitions on each side.

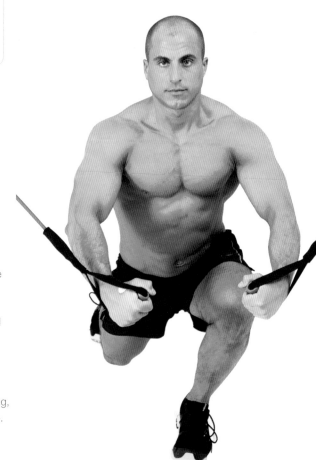

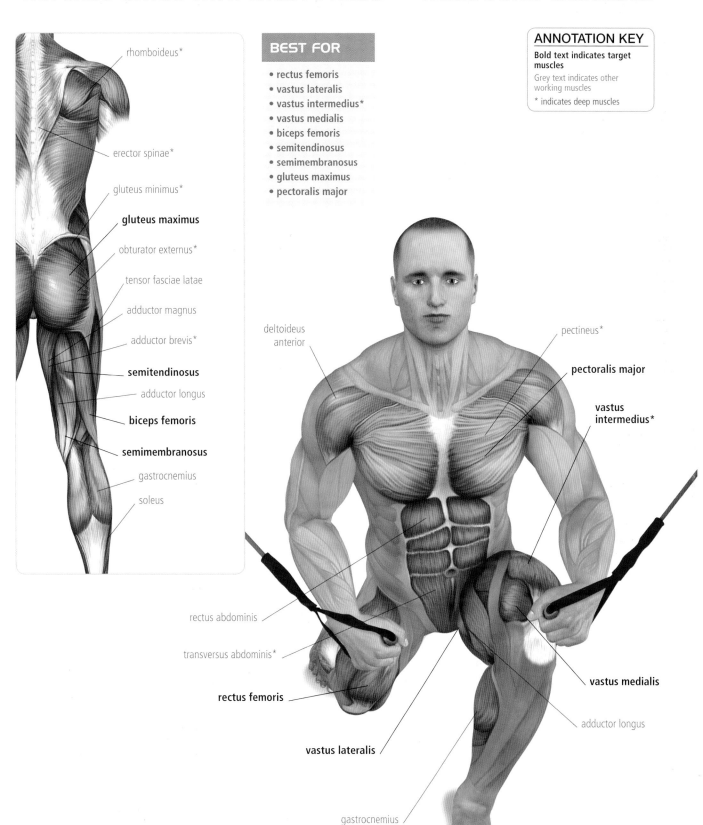

BEST FOR

- rectus femoris
- vastus lateralis
- vastus intermedius*
- vastus medialis
- biceps femoris
- semitendinosus
- semimembranosus
- gluteus maximus
- pectoralis major

ANNOTATION KEY

Bold text indicates target muscles

Grey text indicates other working muscles

* indicates deep muscles

rhomboideus*

erector spinae*

gluteus minimus*

gluteus maximus

obturator externus*

tensor fasciae latae

adductor magnus

adductor brevis*

semitendinosus

adductor longus

biceps femoris

semimembranosus

gastrocnemius

soleus

deltoideus anterior

pectineus*

pectoralis major

vastus intermedius*

rectus abdominis

transversus abdominis*

rectus femoris

vastus medialis

adductor longus

vastus lateralis

gastrocnemius

PRESS AND SQUAT

 Loop a resistance band around a weight machine. Stand facing away from the machine, your feet planted hip-distance apart or slightly wider, and grasp one handle in each hand.

2 Bend your elbows, feeling resistance from the band as you raise both handles to shoulder height.

AVOID
- Locking your knees.
- Arching your back.
- Letting your neck twist.
- Twisting your torso to either side.

BENEFITS
- Strengthens and tones arms, core and gluteal muscles

PERFORMANCE BOOST
- Skiing
- Skating and rollerblading
- Rowing
- All field sports

DO IT RIGHT
- Keep your shoulders pressed down your back.
- Anchor both feet to the floor.
- Keep your torso facing forward and your hips level as you lift and lower.

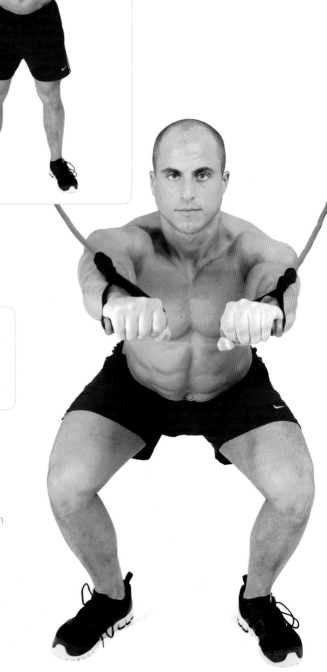

3 Bend your knees into a squat position. Simultaneously straighten both arms in front of you, feeling resistance as you press.

4 Gradually straighten your knees and release the handles, returning your arms to starting position. Perform 15 repetitions.

BEST FOR

- gluteus maximus
- pectoralis major
- rectus femoris
- vastus lateralis
- vastus intermedius*
- vastus medialis
- biceps femoris
- semitendinosus
- semimembranosus

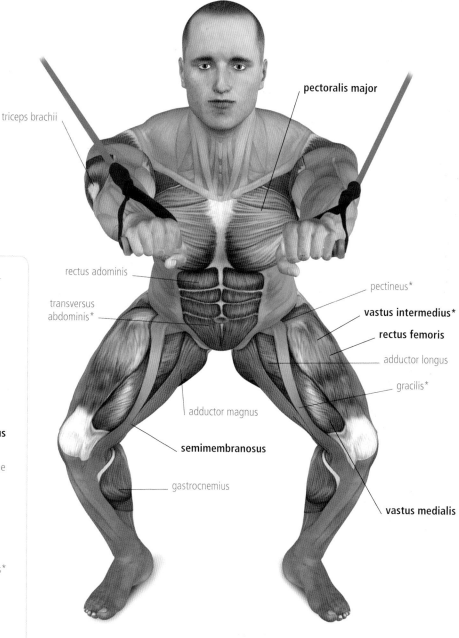

triceps brachii

pectoralis major

rectus adominis

transversus abdominis*

pectineus*

vastus intermedius*

rectus femoris

adductor longus

gracilis*

adductor magnus

semimembranosus

gastrocnemius

vastus medialis

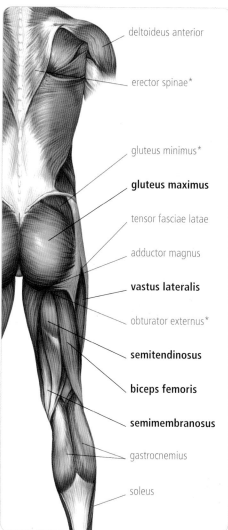

deltoideus anterior

erector spinae*

gluteus minimus*

gluteus maximus

tensor fasciae latae

adductor magnus

vastus lateralis

obturator externus*

semitendinosus

biceps femoris

semimembranosus

gastrocnemius

soleus

ANNOTATION KEY

Bold text indicates target muscles

Grey text indicates other working muscles

* indicates deep muscles

HIP EXTENSION WITH REVERSE FLY

1 Stand upright, facing a cable machine, with your feet less than hip-width apart and a cable attached to your right ankle. Hold one dumbbell in each hand.

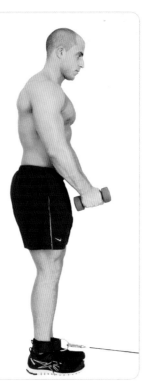

2 Begin to smoothly lift your right leg off the floor. Simultaneously, lift both arms out to your sides. Allow your torso to hinge forward slightly as you lift.

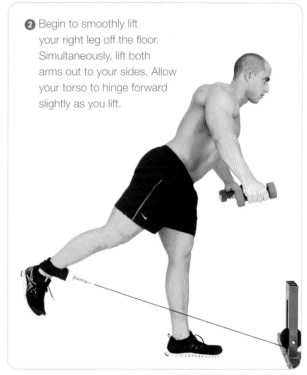

BENEFITS
- Strengthens and tones arms, back and core
- Improves coordination

PERFORMANCE BOOST
- Freeform skiing
- Snowboarding
- Gymnastics
- Tennis
- All field sports

3 Continue to lift your arms and your leg, raising them as high as you can go without arching your back. Your hips should remain stable and facing forward.

4 Gradually lower your right foot to the floor, lower your arms to your sides, and stand upright to return to starting position.

5 Repeat, aiming for 5 repetitions at first. Then, switch the cable to your left ankle and repeat.

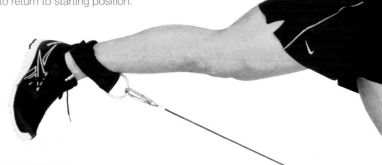

DO IT RIGHT
- Move both of your arms and your weighted leg at roughly the same pace.
- Gaze forward, focusing on a spot in front of you to help with balance.
- Keep your abdominal and gluteal muscles pulled in and engaged.

AVOID
- Rushing through any part of the movement.
- Twisting your hips to either side.
- Hunching your shoulders.
- Letting your neck twist.

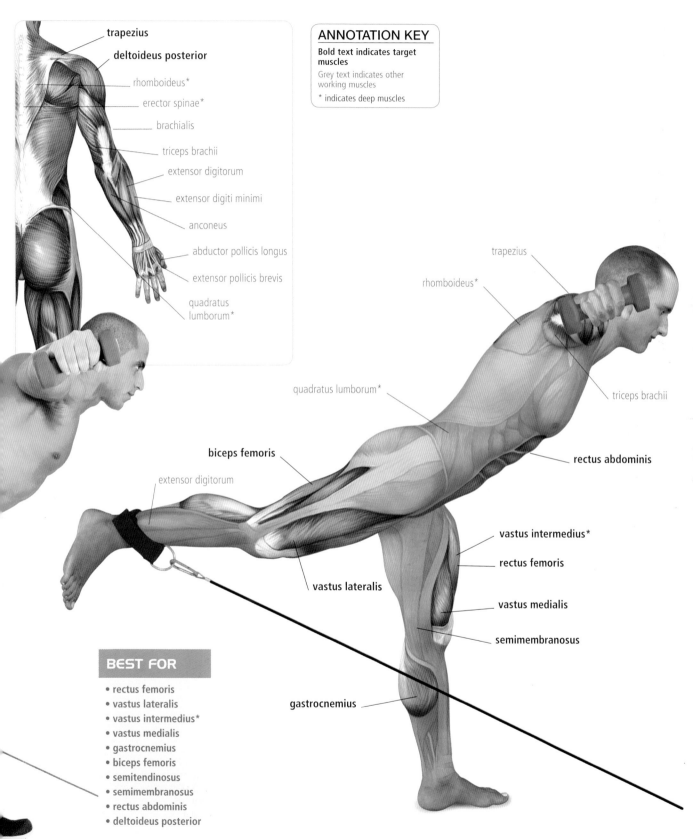

trapezius

deltoideus posterior

rhomboideus*

erector spinae*

brachialis

triceps brachii

extensor digitorum

extensor digiti minimi

anconeus

abductor pollicis longus

extensor pollicis brevis

quadratus lumborum*

ANNOTATION KEY

Bold text indicates target muscles

Grey text indicates other working muscles

* indicates deep muscles

trapezius

rhomboideus*

triceps brachii

quadratus lumborum*

biceps femoris

extensor digitorum

rectus abdominis

vastus intermedius*

rectus femoris

vastus lateralis

vastus medialis

semimembranosus

gastrocnemius

BEST FOR

• rectus femoris
• vastus lateralis
• vastus intermedius*
• vastus medialis
• gastrocnemius
• biceps femoris
• semitendinosus
• semimembranosus
• rectus abdominis
• deltoideus posterior

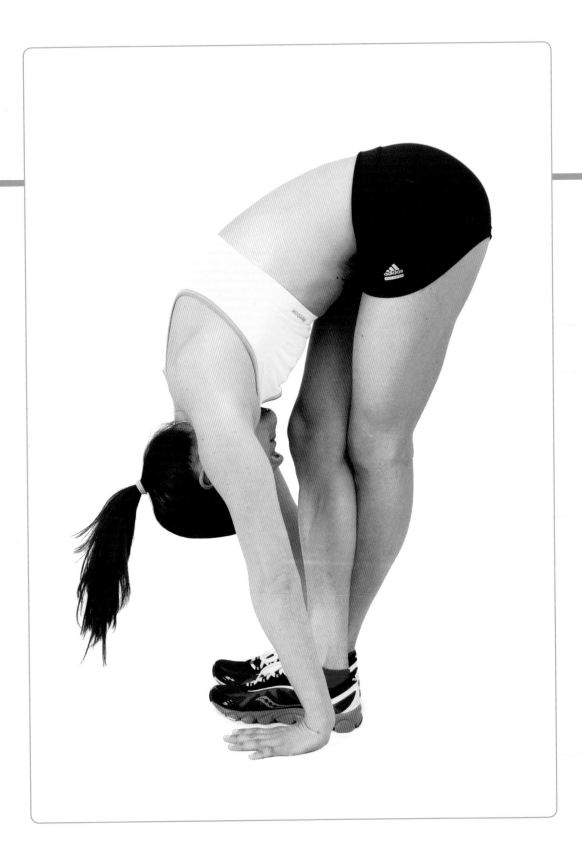

STRETCHING & RELEASING

Stretching and releasing your muscles is vital to your functional regimen. The following exercises will increase your range of motion while releasing stiffness and imbalance from poor posture or overworked muscles. If performed after a workout, they will release fascia (the connective tissue surrounding the muscles) as well as the lactic acid that builds up during exercise. In addition, they will increase circulation and create a feeling of relaxation and wellbeing. Perform them on their own or after an exercise session.

TRICEPS STRETCH

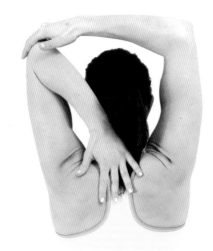

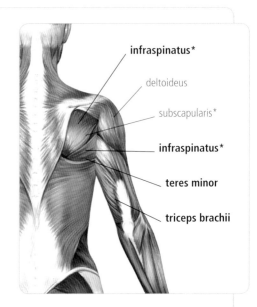

infraspinatus*

deltoideus

subscapularis*

infraspinatus*

teres minor

triceps brachii

BEST FOR

- triceps brachii
- teres minor
- infraspinatus*
- teres major

ANNOTATION KEY
Bold text indicates target muscles
Grey text indicates other working muscles
* indicates deep muscles

BENEFITS
- Stretches and releases stiffness in triceps

PERFORMANCE BOOST
- Baseball
- Tennis

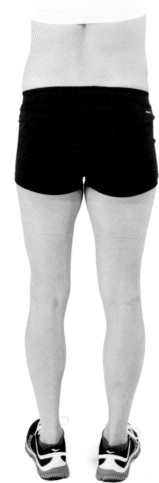

❶ Stand upright, with your arms at your sides. Raise both arms over your head.

❷ Begin to bend both arms. With one hand, grasp the elbow of the other arm and gently pull.

❸ Continue to pull your elbow back until you feel the stretch on the underside of your arm.

❹ Hold for 15 seconds. Release, lowering your arms to your sides. Repeat on the other side. Perform 3 times on each arm.

PECTORAL STRETCH

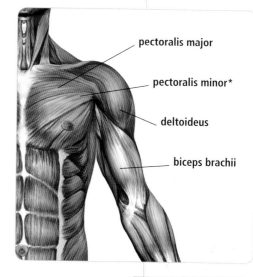

pectoralis major

pectoralis minor*

deltoideus

biceps brachii

BEST FOR

- pectoralis major
- pectoralis minor*
- deltoideus
- biceps brachii

ANNOTATION KEY

Bold text indicates target muscles

Grey text indicates other working muscles

* indicates deep muscles

DO IT RIGHT

- Keep your elbows straight as you move your arms.
- Keep your torso straight and upright.
- To intensify the stretch, try turning your palms outward while lifting your arms.
- Gaze forward.

AVOID

- Leaning your trunk too far forward.
- Turning your head to either side.
- Hunching your shoulders.
- Arching your back excessively.
- Slumping forward.

❶ Stand upright, with your arms at your sides.

❷ Bring your arms behind your back. Clasp your hands together.

❸ Keeping the rest of your body still, imagine your shoulder blades moving toward one another as you lift and reach your clasped hands away from your body.

❹ Hold for 15 seconds. Release, returning to starting position. Repeat 3 times.

BENEFITS

- Stretches and releases stiffness in shoulders, biceps, and chest muscles

PERFORMANCE BOOST

- Baseballl
- Tennis

CALF STRETCH

DO IT RIGHT
- To enhance the stretch, bend your knee more deeply and lower your body further.
- Keep your foot strongly flexed.

AVOID
- Tensing your shoulders.

BEST FOR
- gastrocnemius

BENEFITS
- Stretches calves
- Releases Achilles tendon stiffness

PERFORMANCE BOOST
- Running
- Tennis
- All field sports

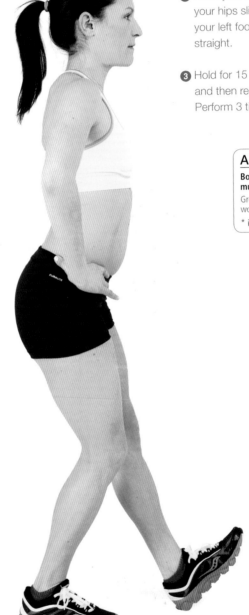

① Stand with your feet parallel and shoulder-width apart. Extend your left leg forward.

② Bend your right knee as you tip your hips slightly forward. Flex your left foot, keeping the left leg straight.

③ Hold for 15 seconds. Release, and then repeat on the other side. Perform 3 times on each leg.

ANNOTATION KEY

Bold text indicates target muscles

Grey text indicates other working muscles

* indicates deep muscles

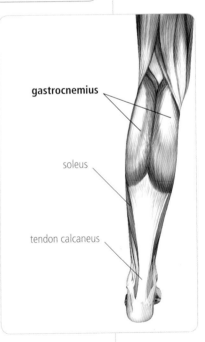

gastrocnemius

soleus

tendon calcaneus

QUADRICEPS STRETCH

1. Stand with your feet together. Bend your left leg behind you, and grasp your foot with your left hand.

2. Pull your heel toward your buttocks until you feel a stretch in the front of your left thigh.

3. Hold for 15 seconds. Release, and then repeat on the other side. Perform 3 times on each leg.

ANNOTATION KEY

Bold text indicates target muscles

Grey text indicates other working muscles

* indicates deep muscles

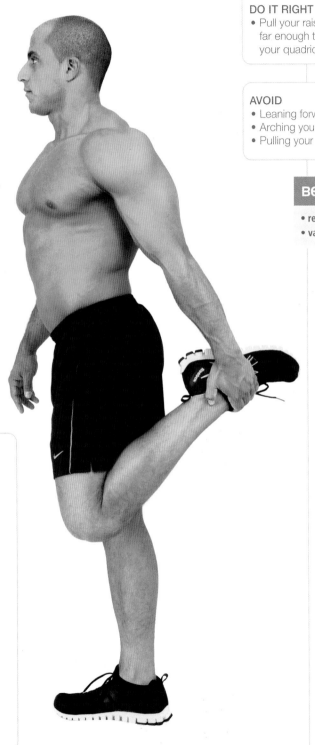

DO IT RIGHT
• Pull your raised knee back far enough to feel a stretch in your quadriceps.

AVOID
• Leaning forward.
• Arching your back.
• Pulling your leg too abruptly.

BEST FOR
• **rectus femoris**
• **vastus medialis**

BENEFITS
• Stretches and releases stiffness in fronts of thighs
• Helps to release lower-back tension

PERFORMANCE BOOST
• Running
• Tennis
• All field sports

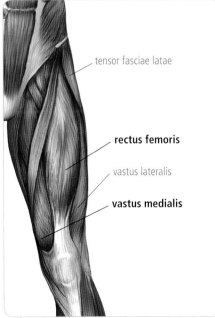

tensor fasciae latae

rectus femoris

vastus lateralis

vastus medialis

PIRIFORMIS STRETCH

❶ Lie on your back, with your legs extended and your arms along your sides. Bend your knees.

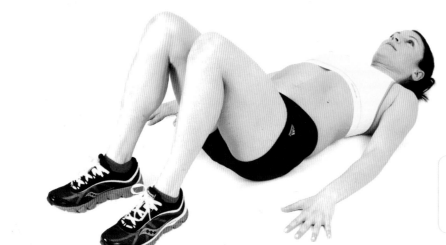

DO IT RIGHT
- Relax your hips to enable a deeper stretch.
- Perform the stretch slowly.

BENEFITS
- Releases stiffness in hips, piriformis and lower back

PERFORMANCE BOOST
- Running
- Biking
- Skating or rollerblading

❷ Keeping your arms and torso in place, lift both feet off the ground. Bring your right ankle over your left knee, resting it on the thigh.

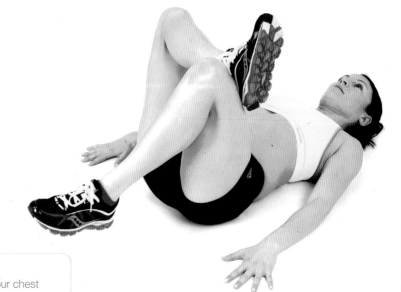

AVOID
- Pulling your thigh to your chest too forcefully, or in a jerky manner.
- Lifting your neck off the floor.

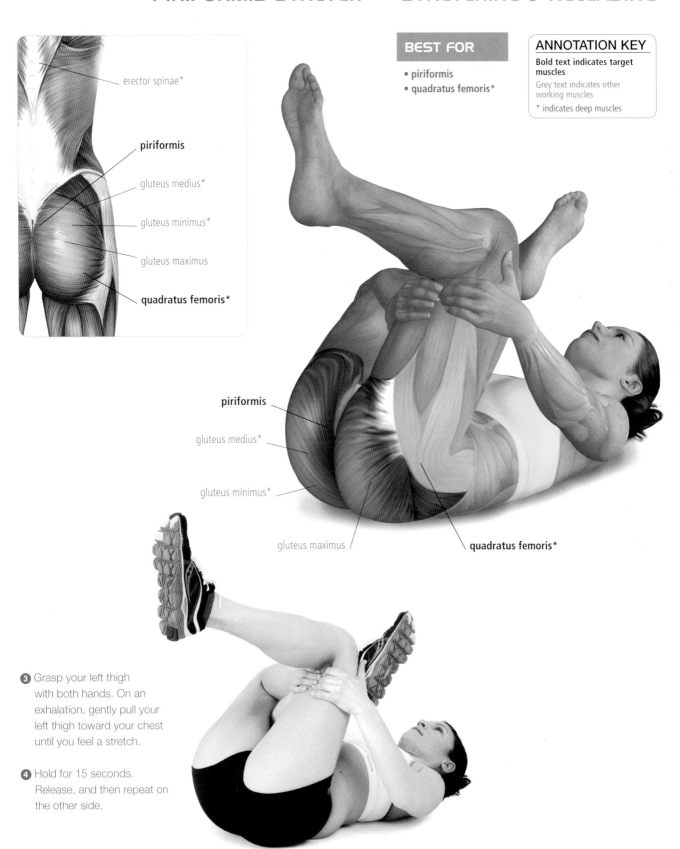

BEST FOR

- piriformis
- quadratus femoris*

ANNOTATION KEY

Bold text indicates target muscles

Grey text indicates other working muscles

* indicates deep muscles

erector spinae*

piriformis

gluteus medius*

gluteus minimus*

gluteus maximus

quadratus femoris*

piriformis

gluteus medius*

gluteus minimus*

gluteus maximus

quadratus femoris*

❸ Grasp your left thigh with both hands. On an exhalation, gently pull your left thigh toward your chest until you feel a stretch.

❹ Hold for 15 seconds. Release, and then repeat on the other side.

HIP-TO-THIGH STRETCH

❶ Kneeling on your right knee, place your left foot in front of you. Your left foot should be flat on the floor, your right heel lifted.

❷ Shift your weight and gradually bring your torso forward, bending your left knee more deeply so that the knee shifts toward your toes.

DO IT RIGHT
- Relax your shoulders and neck.
- Keep your upper body stable.

AVOID
- Performing this exercise if you have groin injury.

BENEFITS
- Stretches hips and thighs
- Improves range of motion in arms and legs

PERFORMANCE BOOST
- Weightlifting
- Skiing
- Skating or rollerblading
- Running

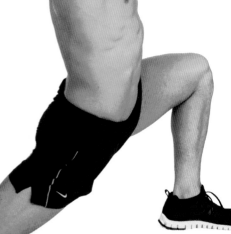

❸ Keeping your torso stable, press your left hip forward until you feel a stretch over the front of your thigh.

❹ Raise your arms toward the ceiling. Hold for 10 seconds, release, and repeat up to 4 more times. Switch sides and repeat.

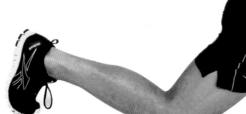

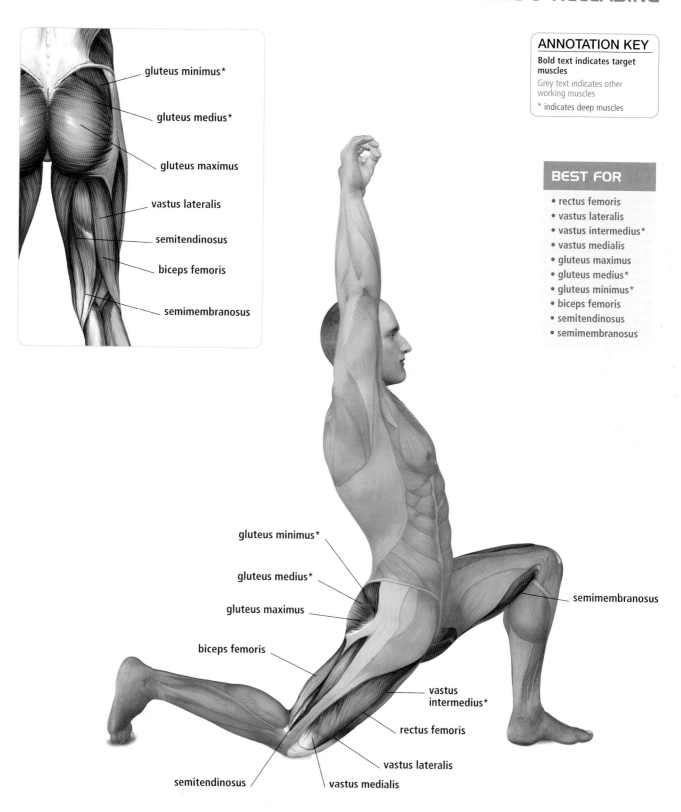

ANNOTATION KEY

Bold text indicates target muscles

Grey text indicates other working muscles

* indicates deep muscles

BEST FOR

- rectus femoris
- vastus lateralis
- vastus intermedius*
- vastus medialis
- gluteus maximus
- gluteus medius*
- gluteus minimus*
- biceps femoris
- semitendinosus
- semimembranosus

gluteus minimus*

gluteus medius*

gluteus maximus

vastus lateralis

semitendinosus

biceps femoris

semimembranosus

gluteus minimus*

gluteus medius*

gluteus maximus

biceps femoris

semimembranosus

vastus intermedius*

rectus femoris

vastus lateralis

semitendinosus

vastus medialis

NECK FLEXION

ANNOTATION KEY

Bold text indicates target muscles

Grey text indicates other working muscles

* indicates deep muscles

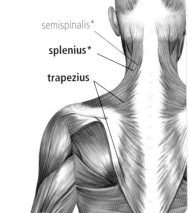

semispinalis*

splenius*

trapezius

DO IT RIGHT
- Keep one arm at your side.
- Let your gaze fall forward.
- Stretch gently.
- Keep your back straight.

BEST FOR

- **splenius***
- **trapezius***

AVOID
- Hunching your shoulders.
- Pulling your head forward so forcefully that the stretch feels uncomfortable.

BENEFITS
- Stretches neck

PERFORMANCE BOOST
- Counteracts neck strain after using a computer or driving for long periods

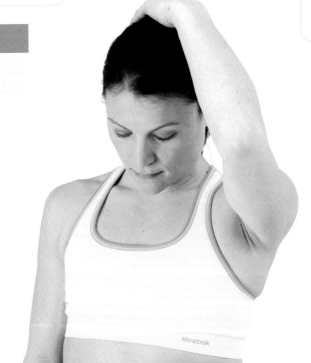

❶ Stand upright. Place one hand on your head. Gradually pull your chin toward your chest until you feel a stretch in the back of your neck.

❷ Hold for 15 seconds. Release and repeat 2 more times. Switch sides and repeat.

NECK SIDE BEND

ANNOTATION KEY

Bold text indicates target muscles

Grey text indicates other working muscles

* indicates deep muscles

scalenus*

trapezius

sternocleidomastoideus

AVOID
• Hunching your shoulders.
• Pulling your head too abruptly to the side.

DO IT RIGHT
• Gaze forward.
• Stretch gently.
• Keep your back straight.

BEST FOR
• sternoclei-domastoideus
• trapezius
• scalenus*

BENEFITS
• Releases stiffness in sides of neck

PERFORMANCE BOOST
• Counteracts neck strain after using a computer or driving for long periods

❶ Stand upright. Gently grasp the side of your head with one hand.

❷ Reach toward the small of the back with your other hand, bending at the elbw.

❸ Tilt your head toward your raised elbow until you feel a stretch in the side of your neck.

❹ Hold for 15 seconds. Release and repeat 2 more times. Switch sides and repeat.

ILIOTIBIAL BAND STRETCH

❶ Stand upright, with your arms along your sides. Cross one foot in front of the other.

DO IT RIGHT
- Keep your knees straight (yet soft) throughout the exercise.
- Let your head drop.

AVOID
- Bending or locking your knees.
- Twisting your neck, shoulders or torso to either side.

❷ Bending at your waist, gradually reach toward the floor with your hands.

❸ Hold for 15 seconds. Release, slowly roll up, and repeat twice. Switch sides and repeat.

BENEFITS
- Stretches IT band
- Counteracts effects of wearing high heels

PERFORMANCE BOOST
- Skiing
- Running
- Biking

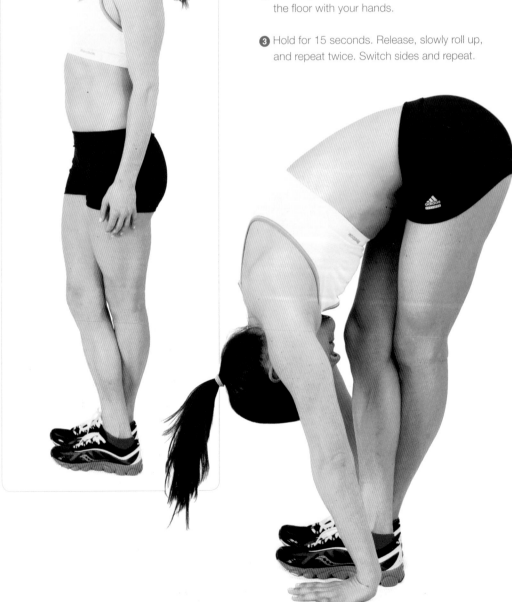

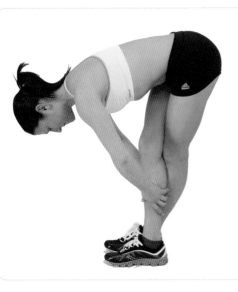

MODIFICATION

Easier: If you find it difficult to reach the floor with your hands while maintaining your form, hold the stretch when your hands are only partway to the floor. Try to reach slightly lower each time you stretch.

ANNOTATION KEY

Bold text indicates target muscles

Grey text indicates other working muscles

* indicates deep muscles

BEST FOR

- **gluteus maximus**
- **semitendinosus**
- **biceps femoris**
- **tractus iliotibialis**

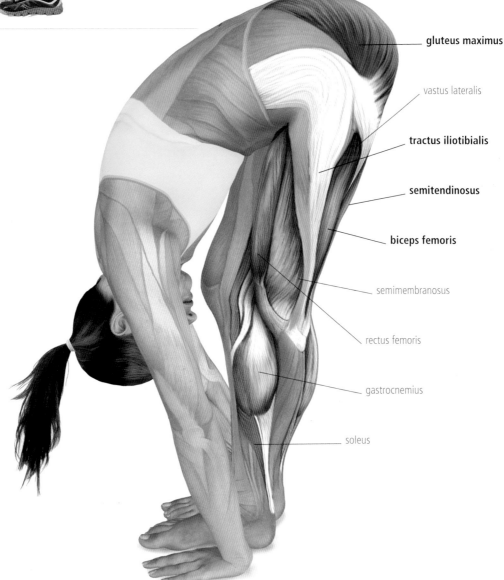

gluteus maximus

vastus lateralis

tractus iliotibialis

semitendinosus

biceps femoris

semimembranosus

rectus femoris

gastrocnemius

soleus

SUPINE HAMSTRINGS STRETCH

❶ Lie on your back with both knees bent and your feet flat on the floor.

❷ Using both hands, grasp one leg just above the knee.

❸ Gradually draw your knee toward your chest.

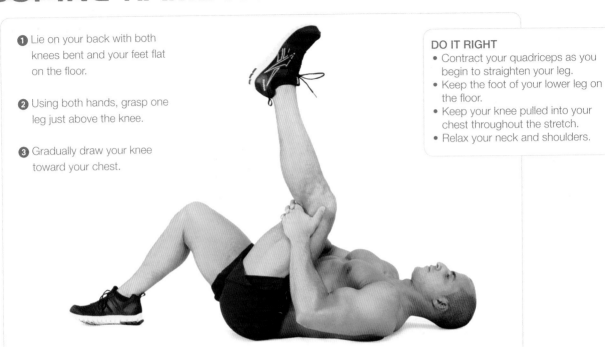

DO IT RIGHT
- Contract your quadriceps as you begin to straighten your leg.
- Keep the foot of your lower leg on the floor.
- Keep your knee pulled into your chest throughout the stretch.
- Relax your neck and shoulders.

AVOID
- Lifting your head.
- Rounding your shoulders.
- Letting your stabilising leg shift to either side.

BENEFITS
- Stretches hamstrings
- Helps to prevent lower-back pain

PERFORMANCE BOOST
- All field sports

❹ Keeping the knee in place, begin to straighten the leg. Your toe should be flexed.

❺ Release your leg into the stretch. Maintaining your form, pull the leg toward your chest.

❻ Let go of the leg, return to starting position, and repeat on the other side. Perform up to 10 times per leg.

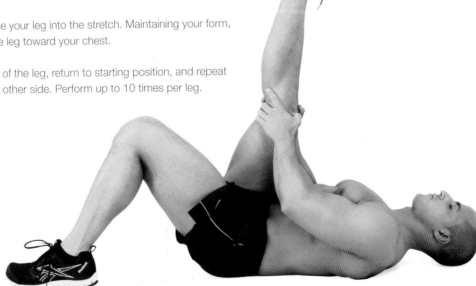

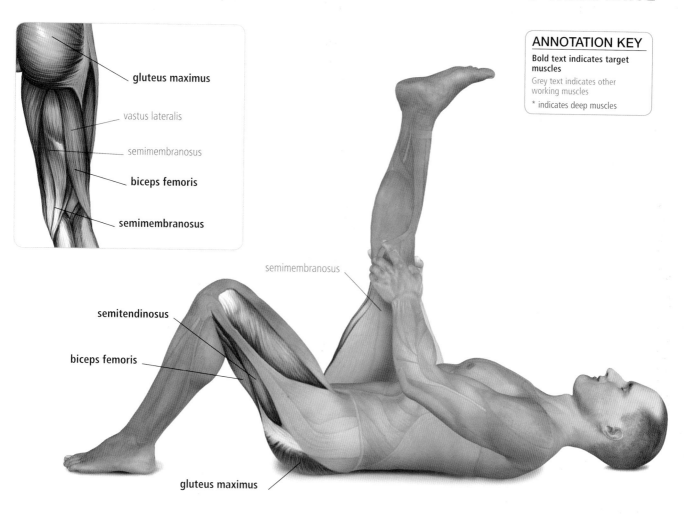

gluteus maximus

vastus lateralis

semimembranosus

biceps femoris

semimembranosus

semimembranosus

semitendinosus

biceps femoris

gluteus maximus

ANNOTATION KEY

Bold text indicates target muscles

Grey text indicates other working muscles

* indicates deep muscles

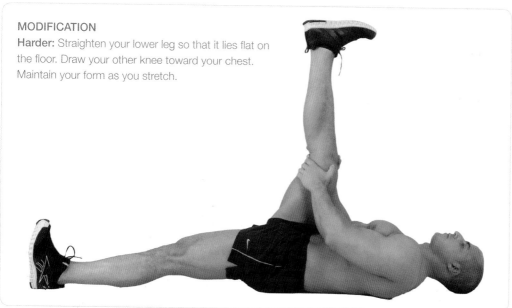

MODIFICATION

Harder: Straighten your lower leg so that it lies flat on the floor. Draw your other knee toward your chest. Maintain your form as you stretch.

BEST FOR

- gluteus maximus
- semitendinosus
- biceps femoris

SIDE ADDUCTOR STRETCH

❶ Stand upright. Separate your feet until they are wider than hip-distance apart, toes turned slightly outward. If desired, rest your hands just above your knees.

❷ Keeping your torso steady, gradually bend your knees.

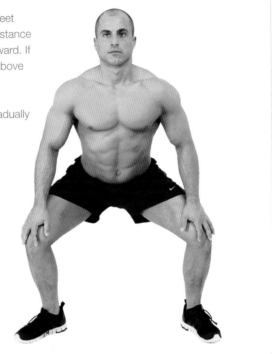

DO IT RIGHT
- Keep your spine neutral and your torso facing forward.
- Let your shoulders come slightly forward as you stretch.
- Anchor your feet to the floor.
- Gaze forward.

BENEFITS
- Stretches side adductors

PERFORMANCE BOOST
- Running
- Skiing
- Tennis

AVOID
- Rounding your spine.
- Hunching your shoulders.
- Tensing your neck.
- Letting either foot lift off the floor.
- Allowing your knees to extend over your toes as you bend.

❸ Without moving your torso, shift your weight to one side, bending your knee while straightening and extending your opposite leg.

❹ Hold, aiming for 10 seconds. Release, return to starting position, and then repeat on the other side.

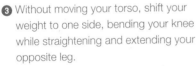
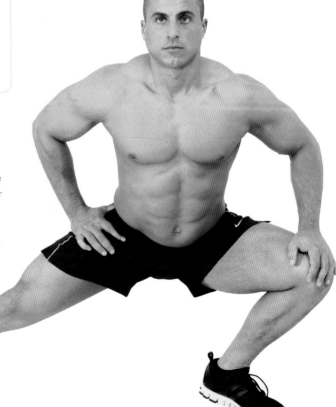

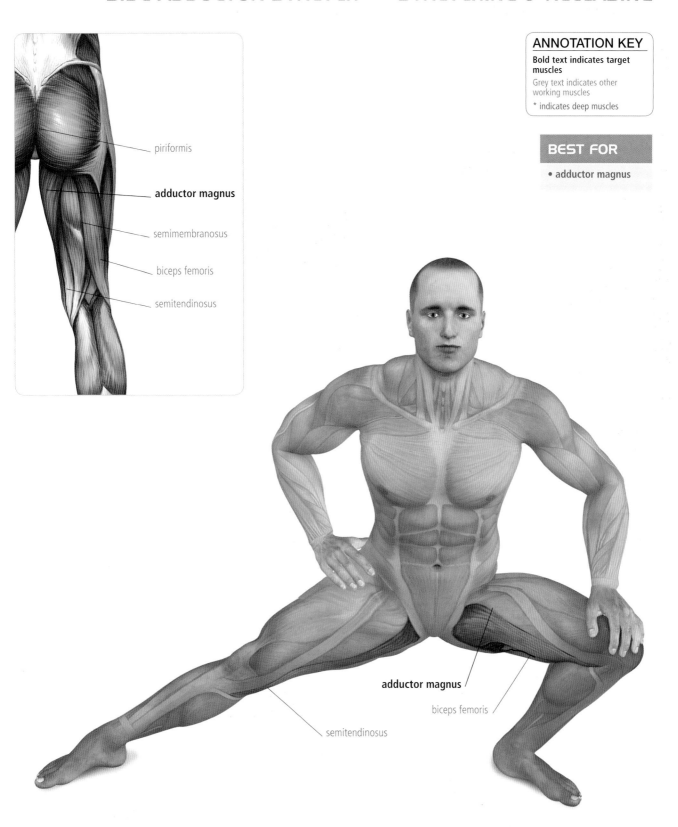

ANNOTATION KEY

Bold text indicates target muscles

Grey text indicates other working muscles

* indicates deep muscles

BEST FOR

• adductor magnus

piriformis

adductor magnus

semimembranosus

biceps femoris

semitendinosus

adductor magnus

biceps femoris

semitendinosus

COBRA STRETCH

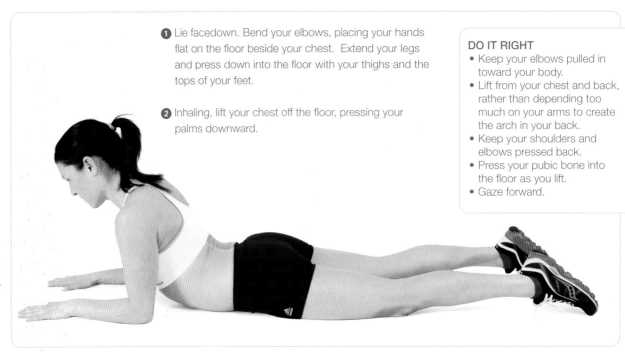

1 Lie facedown. Bend your elbows, placing your hands flat on the floor beside your chest. Extend your legs and press down into the floor with your thighs and the tops of your feet.

2 Inhaling, lift your chest off the floor, pressing your palms downward.

DO IT RIGHT
- Keep your elbows pulled in toward your body.
- Lift from your chest and back, rather than depending too much on your arms to create the arch in your back.
- Keep your shoulders and elbows pressed back.
- Press your pubic bone into the floor as you lift.
- Gaze forward.

AVOID
- Tensing your buttocks.
- Splaying your elbows out to the sides.
- Lifting your hips off the floor.
- Twisting your neck.

BENEFITS
- Strengthens spine and gluteal muscles
- Stretches chest, abdominals and shoulders

PERFORMANCE BOOST
- All sports

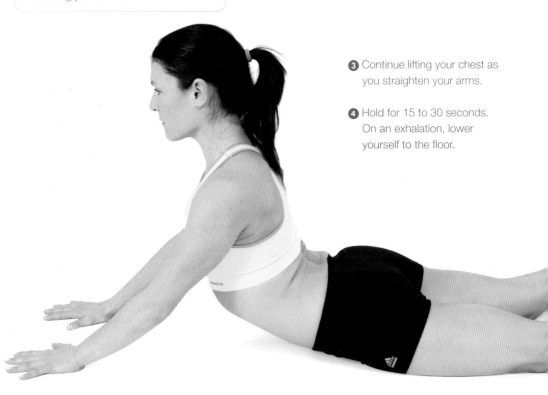

3 Continue lifting your chest as you straighten your arms.

4 Hold for 15 to 30 seconds. On an exhalation, lower yourself to the floor.

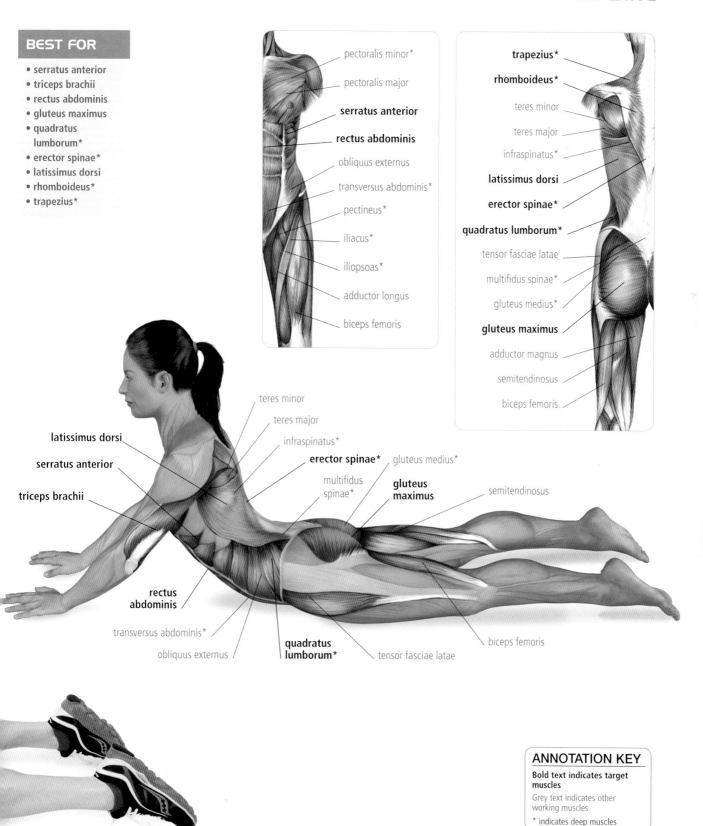

BEST FOR

- serratus anterior
- triceps brachii
- rectus abdominis
- gluteus maximus
- quadratus lumborum*
- erector spinae*
- latissimus dorsi
- rhomboideus*
- trapezius*

pectoralis minor*

pectoralis major

serratus anterior

rectus abdominis

obliquus externus

transversus abdominis*

pectineus*

iliacus*

iliopsoas*

adductor longus

biceps femoris

trapezius*

rhomboideus*

teres minor

teres major

infraspinatus*

latissimus dorsi

erector spinae*

quadratus lumborum*

tensor fasciae latae

multifidus spinae*

gluteus medius*

gluteus maximus

adductor magnus

semitendinosus

biceps femoris

latissimus dorsi

serratus anterior

triceps brachii

teres minor

teres major

infraspinatus*

erector spinae*

gluteus medius*

multifidus spinae*

gluteus maximus

semitendinosus

rectus abdominis

transversus abdominis*

obliquus externus

quadratus lumborum*

tensor fasciae latae

biceps femoris

ANNOTATION KEY

Bold text indicates target muscles

Grey text indicates other working muscles

* indicates deep muscles

KNEELING SIDE LIFT

1 Kneel on the floor, with your left leg outstretched to the side and your right leg lined up under your hips. Place both hands behind your head, with your elbows pointing out to the sides.

2 Begin leaning your torso to the right.

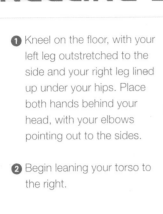

DO IT RIGHT
- Relax and lengthen your neck.
- Elongate your leg as much as possible.
- Lift your leg only as high as you can go without affecting your form.
- Keep your abs, especially the obliques, strongly engaged.

BENEFITS
- Tones abdominal muscles

PERFORMANCE BOOST
- All field sports

AVOID
- Twisting your torso.
- Hunching your shoulders.
- Arching your back or hunching forward.
- Tensing your neck.

3 Lift your left leg off the floor, bringing it as high as your hips.

4 Lower your leg. Repeat 3 to 5 times. Then, switch sides and repeat.

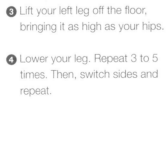

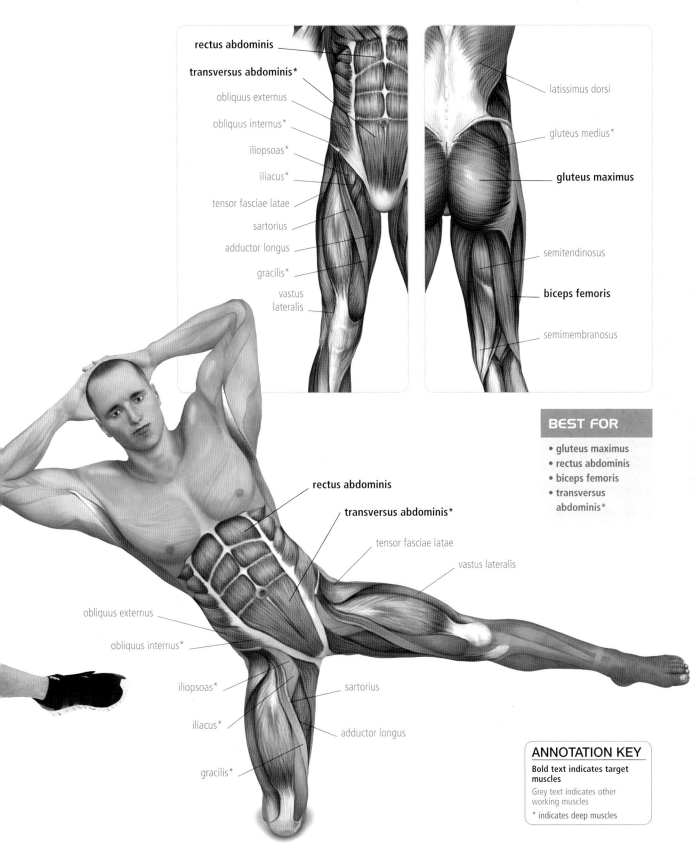

rectus abdominis

transversus abdominis*

obliquus externus

obliquus internus*

iliopsoas*

iliacus*

tensor fasciae latae

sartorius

adductor longus

gracilis*

vastus lateralis

latissimus dorsi

gluteus medius*

gluteus maximus

semitendinosus

biceps femoris

semimembranosus

rectus abdominis

transversus abdominis*

tensor fasciae latae

vastus lateralis

obliquus externus

obliquus internus*

iliopsoas*

iliacus*

sartorius

adductor longus

gracilis*

BEST FOR

- gluteus maximus
- rectus abdominis
- biceps femoris
- transversus abdominis*

ANNOTATION KEY

Bold text indicates target muscles

Grey text indicates other working muscles

* indicates deep muscles

QUADRICEPS ROLL

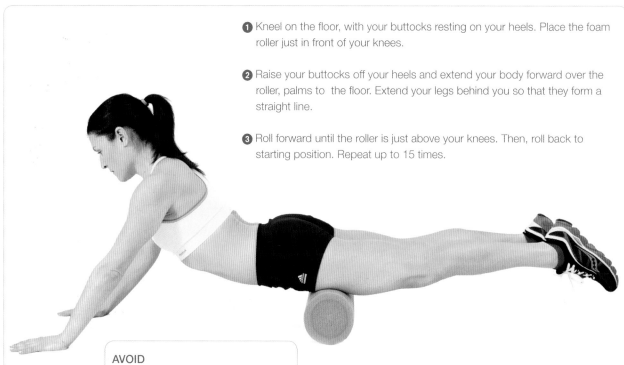

❶ Kneel on the floor, with your buttocks resting on your heels. Place the foam roller just in front of your knees.

❷ Raise your buttocks off your heels and extend your body forward over the roller, palms to the floor. Extend your legs behind you so that they form a straight line.

❸ Roll forward until the roller is just above your knees. Then, roll back to starting position. Repeat up to 15 times.

AVOID
- Turning your neck.
- Twisting your torso to either side.

BENEFITS
- Releases fascia
- Improves range of motion
- Relieves quadriceps stiffness

PERFORMANCE BOOST
- All activities

DO IT RIGHT
- Press your palms into the floor as you roll back and forth.
- Point your toes.
- Pull in your abdominal muscles.
- Keep your palms anchored.
- Gaze towards the floor.

rectus abdominus

vastus intermedius*

rectus femoris

vastus lateralis

vastus medialis

BEST FOR
- rectus femoris
- vastus lateralis
- vastus intermedius*
- vastus medialis

ANNOTATION KEY
Bold text indicates target muscles
Grey text indicates other working muscles
* indicates deep muscles

HAMSTRINGS ROLL

❶ Sit on the floor, resting your palms behind you. Position the foam roller beneath your thighs, just above the knees. Extend both legs, heels slightly off the floor.

❷ Pushing forward with your arms, roll forward until the foam roller is below the uppermost part of the backs of your thighs.

❸ Roll back to starting position. Repeat up to 15 times.

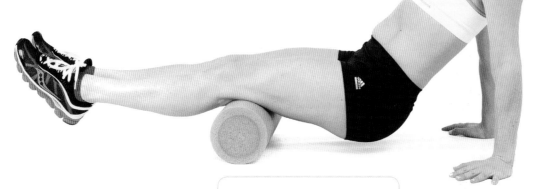

DO IT RIGHT
- Press your palms into the floor.
- Keep your arms and abs strongly engaged.
- Gaze forward.
- Keep both legs extended while rolling.

AVOID
- Positioning the foam roller at your knee.
- Letting your belly bulge outward.
- Twisting your hips to either side.
- Letting your palms come off the floor.

BENEFITS
- Relieves tightness in hamstrings
- Improves range of motion

PERFORMANCE BOOST
- All activities

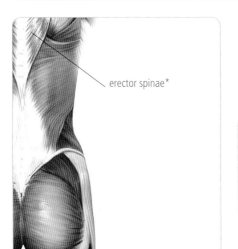

erector spinae*

semitendinosus

biceps femoris

semimembranosus

ANNOTATION KEY
Bold text indicates target muscles

Grey text indicates other working muscles

* indicates deep muscles

BEST FOR
- biceps femoris
- semitendinosus
- semimembranosus

GLUTEAL ROLL

❶ Sit on the floor, resting your palms on the floor behind you. Position the foam roller beneath the upper part of your buttocks. Extend both legs, resting your heels on the floor.

❷ In a controlled movement, roll slightly back until the roller is beneath the lower part of your buttocks.

❸ Return to starting position. Repeat, performing 10 repetitions.

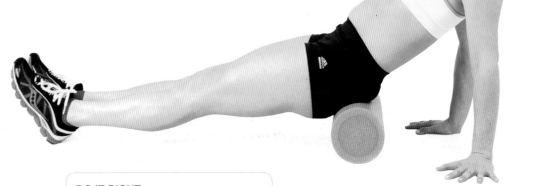

DO IT RIGHT
- Move smoothly.
- Keep your arms and abs strongly engaged.
- Press your palms into the floor.
- Gaze forward.

AVOID
- Arching your back.
- Twisting your torso.
- Letting your palms come off the floor.

BENEFITS
- Relieves tightness in gluteal muscles, especially useful after sitting for long periods
- Improves range of motion

PERFORMANCE BOOST
- All activities

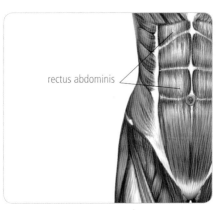

rectus abdominis

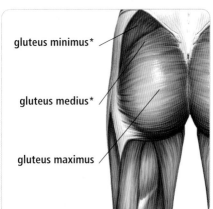

gluteus minimus*

gluteus medius*

gluteus maximus

BEST FOR
- gluteus maximus
- gluteus medius*
- gluteus minimus*

ANNOTATION KEY
Bold text indicates target muscles
Grey text indicates other working muscles
* indicates deep muscles

LATISSIMUS ROLL

❶ Lie on your right side, with the foam roller below the side of your upper chest and your legs extended. Support your torso by placing your right forearm on the floor.

❷ Bend your left leg and cross it in front of your right, placing your left foot on the floor.

❸ Pushing into the floor with your left leg, roll forward so that the roller moves down the side of your torso.

❹ Smoothly roll back to starting position. Repeat, completing 5 repetitions. Switch sides and repeat.

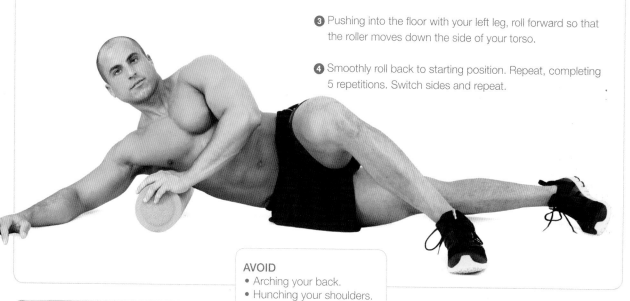

AVOID
- Arching your back.
- Hunching your shoulders.
- Tensing your neck.

DO IT RIGHT
- Move smoothly.
- Keep your abs engaged.
- Press your forearm into the floor.
- Press your shoulders down toward your back.
- Gaze forward.

BENEFITS
- Relieves tightness in lats
- Improves range of motion
- Strengthens scapular stabilisers and lateral trunk muscles

PERFORMANCE BOOST
- All activities

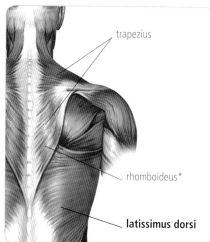

trapezius

rhomboideus*

latissimus dorsi

serratus anterior

rectus abdominis

obliquus externus

obliquus internus*

BEST FOR
- latissimus dorsi

ANNOTATION KEY

Bold text indicates target muscles

Grey text indicates other working muscles

* indicates deep muscles

TENSOR FASCIAE LATAE ROLL

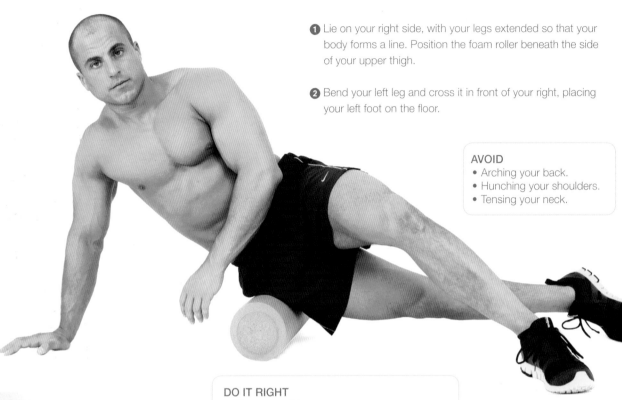

❶ Lie on your right side, with your legs extended so that your body forms a line. Position the foam roller beneath the side of your upper thigh.

❷ Bend your left leg and cross it in front of your right, placing your left foot on the floor.

AVOID
- Arching your back.
- Hunching your shoulders.
- Tensing your neck.

BENEFITS
- Relieves soreness in tensor fasciae latae
- Improves range of motion
- Strengthens scapular stabilisers and lateral trunk muscles

PERFORMANCE BOOST
- All activities

DO IT RIGHT
- Move smoothly.
- Keep your abs engaged.
- Press your palm into the floor.
- Press your shoulders down toward your back.
- Gaze forward.

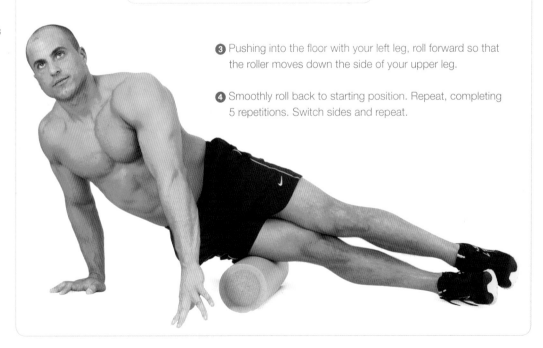

❸ Pushing into the floor with your left leg, roll forward so that the roller moves down the side of your upper leg.

❹ Smoothly roll back to starting position. Repeat, completing 5 repetitions. Switch sides and repeat.

ANNOTATION KEY

Bold text indicates target muscles

Grey text indicates other working muscles

* indicates deep muscles

BEST FOR

• tensor fasciae latae

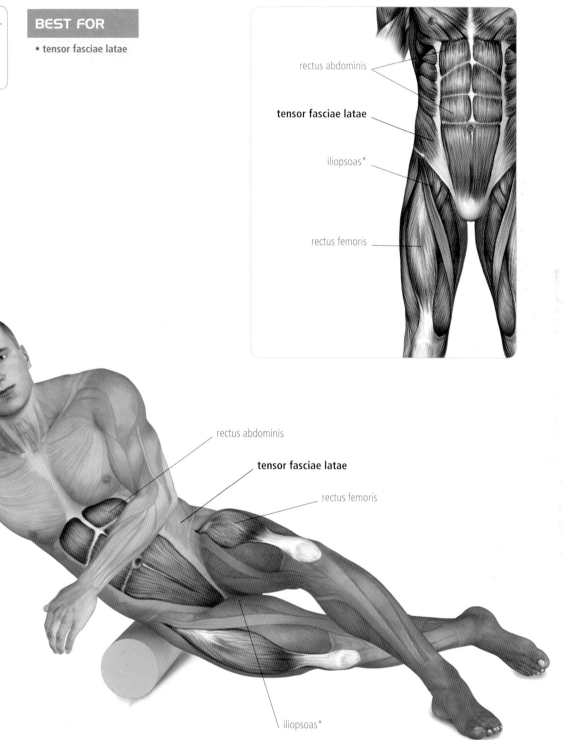

rectus abdominis

tensor fasciae latae

iliopsoas*

rectus femoris

rectus abdominis

tensor fasciae latae

rectus femoris

iliopsoas*

BACK ROLL

❶ Sit with your legs bent, extended in front of you, and your arms at your sides, palms on the floor. Position the foam roller behind you.

AVOID
- Arching your back.
- Hunching your shoulders.
- Tensing your neck.

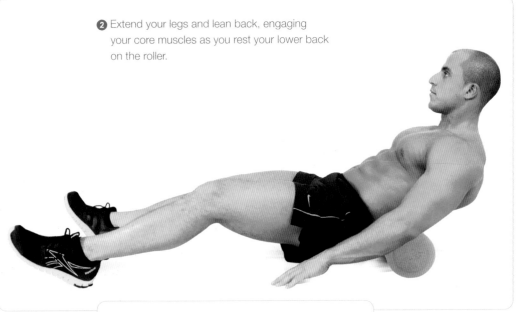

BENEFITS
- Relieves soreness throughout back
- Improves range of motion

PERFORMANCE BOOST
- All activities

❷ Extend your legs and lean back, engaging your core muscles as you rest your lower back on the roller.

DO IT RIGHT
- Move smoothly and with control.
- Use your arms, legs and abs to drive the movement.
- Press your palms into the floor.
- Press your shoulders down toward your back.
- Gaze forward.

3 Gradually roll forward until the roller is beneath your upper back.

4 Roll back to starting position. Repeat, completing 5 repetitions. Then, complete 5 more if desired.

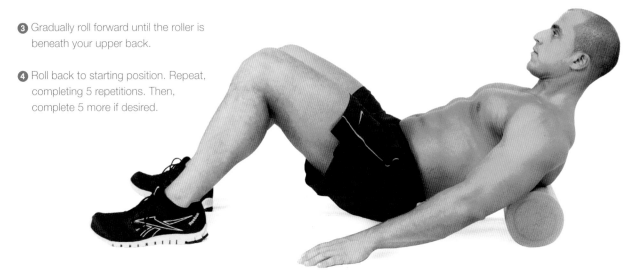

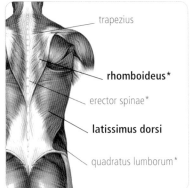

- trapezius
- **rhomboideus***
- erector spinae*
- **latissimus dorsi**
- quadratus lumborum*

BEST FOR

- latissimus dorsi
- rhomboideus*

ANNOTATION KEY

Bold text indicates target muscles

Grey text indicates other working muscles

* indicates deep muscles

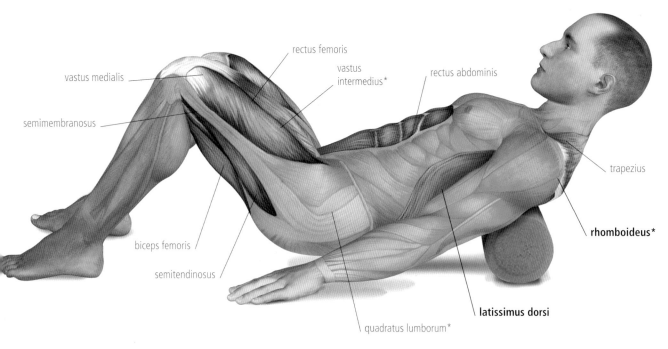

- vastus medialis
- semimembranosus
- rectus femoris
- vastus intermedius*
- rectus abdominis
- trapezius
- **rhomboideus***
- biceps femoris
- semitendinosus
- **latissimus dorsi**
- quadratus lumborum*

THREAD THE NEEDLE

❶ Sit upright with your hands on the floor by your sides, palms down. Place the foam roller beneath your knees.

❷ Keeping your legs firm, press into the floor as you slowly raise your hips until they are level with your knees.

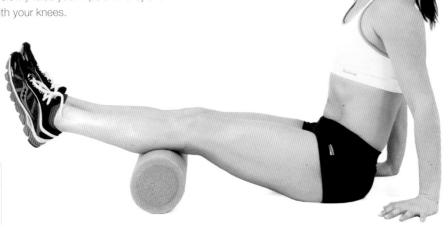

DO IT RIGHT
- Keep your torso upright and facing forward.
- Keep your abdominal muscles engaged.

AVOID
- Twisting to either side.
- Letting your abs bulge outward.
- Twisting your neck.
- Keep your arms anchored to the floor, as stable as possible.
- Performing this exercise if you have wrist or shoulder pain.

BENEFITS
- Stabilises core, pelvis and shoulders
- Strengthens triceps and core muscles

PERFORMANCE BOOST
- All sports, especially those requiring balance

❸ Draw your hips backward through your arms, rolling your legs over the roller. Drop your head slightly so that your gaze is directed toward your thighs.

❹ Moving slowly and with control, roll back to the starting position. Keep your hips lifted off the floor. Repeat, aiming for 15 repetitions.

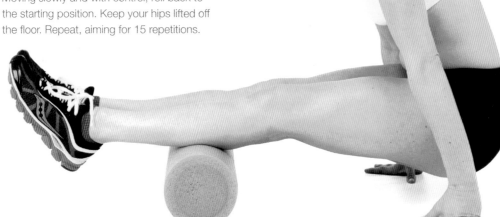

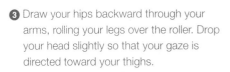

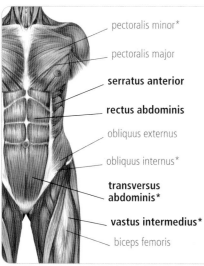

pectoralis minor*

pectoralis major

serratus anterior

rectus abdominis

obliquus externus

obliquus internus*

transversus abdominis*

vastus intermedius*

biceps femoris

BEST FOR

- tensor fasciae latae*
- serratus anterior
- deltoideus
- rectus abdominis
- transversus abdominis*
- vastus intermedius*

ANNOTATION KEY

Bold text indicates target muscles

Grey text indicates other working muscles

* indicates deep muscles

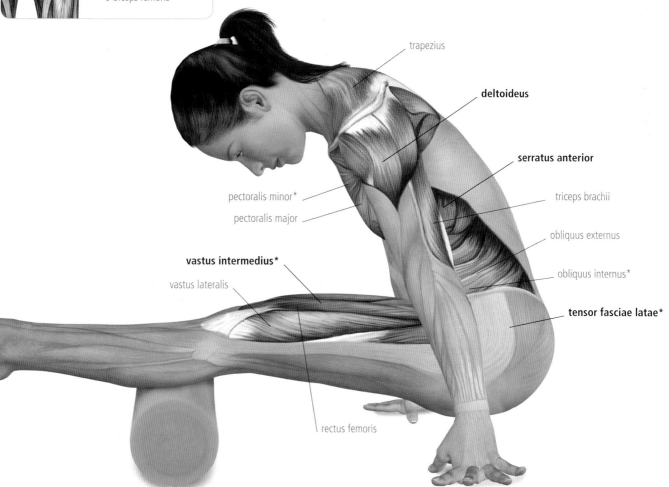

trapezius

deltoideus

serratus anterior

triceps brachii

pectoralis minor*

pectoralis major

obliquus externus

obliquus internus*

tensor fasciae latae*

vastus intermedius*

vastus lateralis

rectus femoris

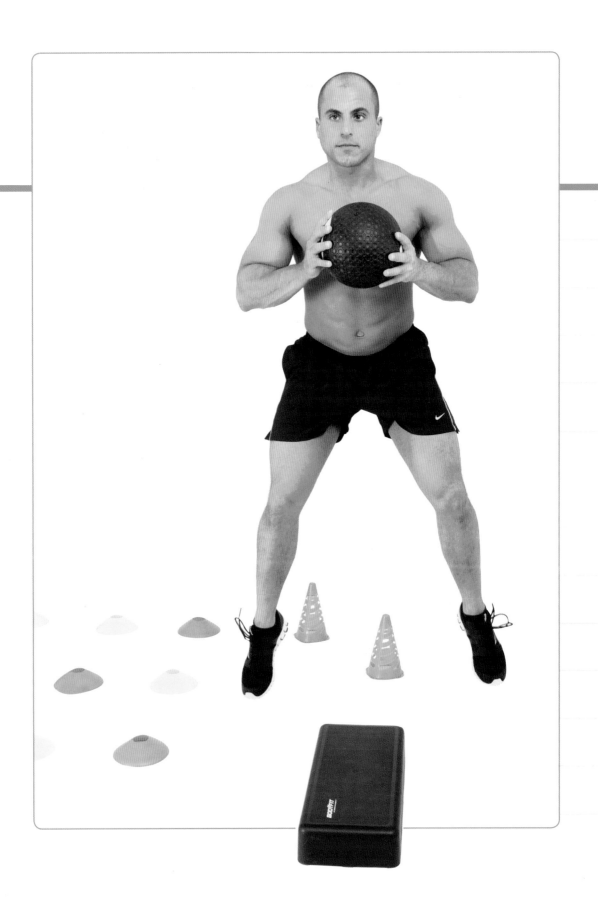

YOUR FUNCTIONAL WORKOUTS

Now that you've gained familiarity with the exercises in this book, try putting them together to form combinations that can function within your daily routine. When your alarm goes off at the crack of dawn, but you'd rather just crawl back into bed, start with Body Blitz. And when you're running to catch the train home – maybe shouldering a giant work bag, maybe balancing in high heels – take comfort in the Tension Buster you can complete when the day is done. From head to toe, you'll feel the benefits of these targeted routines.

BODY BLITZ

This challenging workout will give you a burst of energy, burning calories in the process. Keep your pace up as you move through the exercises.

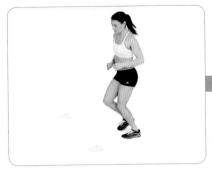

1 Warm-Up Obstacle Course, page 20

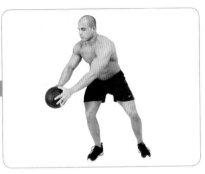

2 Figure 8, page 76

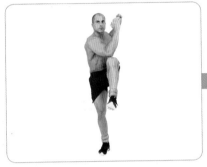

3 Twisting Knee Raise, page 48

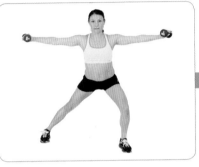

4 Lateral-Extension Lateral Lunge, page 72

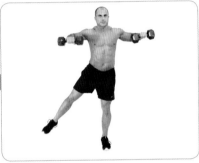

5 Knee Raise with Lateral Extension, page 78

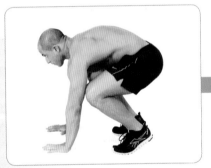

6 Functional Burpee, page 32

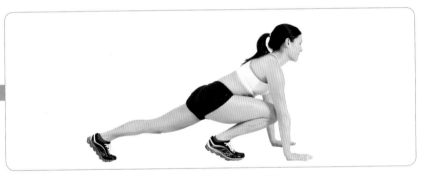

7 Mountain Climber, page 34

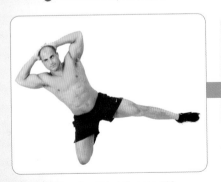

8 Kneeling Side Lift, page 132

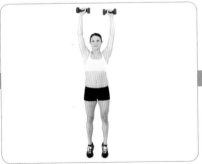

9 Toe Raise with Overhead Press, page 70

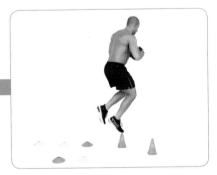

10 Obstacle Challenge, page 96

THE CORE OF IT

Imagine your navel pressing toward your spine, relax your shoulders, and engage your glutes as you feel the powerhouse muscles of your core working, strong and functional.

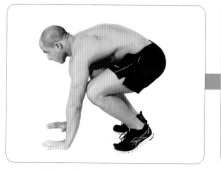

❶ Functional Burpee, page 32

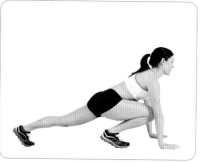

❷ Mountain Climber, page 34

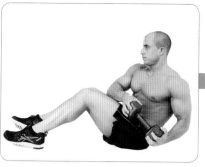

❸ Seated Russian Twist, page 86

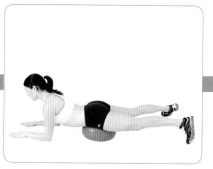

❹ Heel Beat, page 50

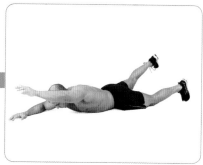

❺ Swimming, page 52

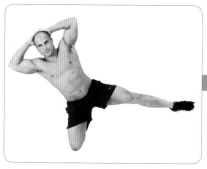

❻ Kneeling Side Lift, page 132

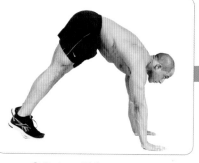

❼ Push-up Walkout, page 44

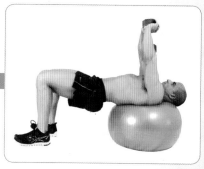

❽ Swiss Ball Pullover, page 88

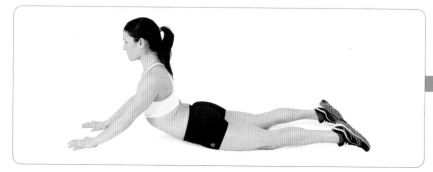

❾ Cobra Stretch, page 130

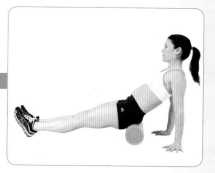

❿ Gluteal Roll, page 136

WORK-TO-PARTY TONER

This routine will tone your arms and the backs of your legs without wiping you out for the evening. At the end, hold your Iliotibial Band Stretch for an extra 10 seconds and then slowly roll up, vertebra by vertebra.

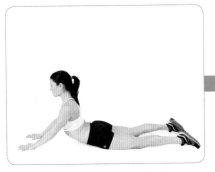

❶ Cobra Stretch, page 130

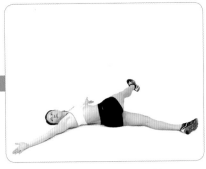

❷ Full-Body Roll, page 60

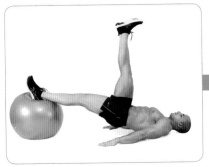

❸ Swiss-Ball Bridging Raise, page 56

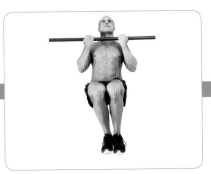

❹ Chin-Up with Hanging Leg Raise, page 58

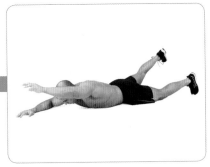

❺ Swimming, page 52

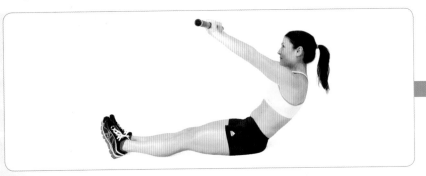

❻ Roll-up Triceps Lift, page 82

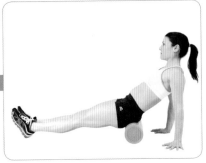

❼ Gluteal Roll, page 136

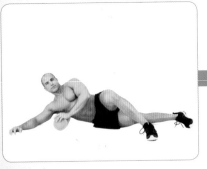

❽ Latissimus Roll, page 137

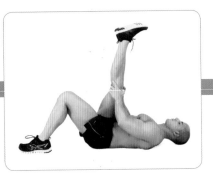

❾ Supine Hamstrings Stretch, page 126

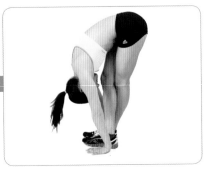

❿ Iliotibial Band Stretch, page 125

LEG INTERLUDE

Practised twice a week, this workout cultivates killer legs — whether you're male or female. Bonus: you can do it at your desk.

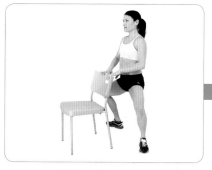

❶ Chair Plié, page 26

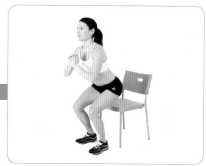

❷ Chair Squat, page 28

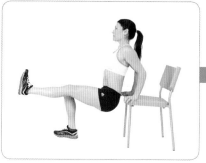

❸ Leg-Extension Chair Dip, page 40

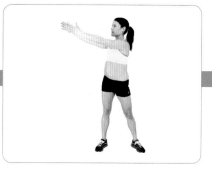

❹ Diagonal Reach, page 22

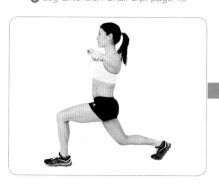

❺ Lateral-Extension Reverse Lunge, page 24

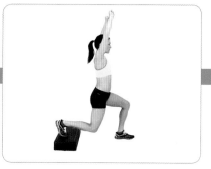

❻ Split Squat with Overhead Reach, page 30

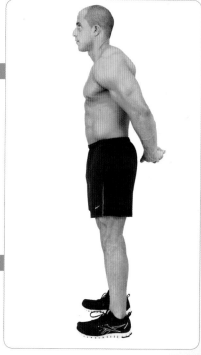

❼ Pectoral Stretch, page 115

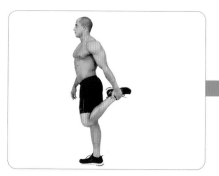

❽ Quadriceps Stretch, page 117

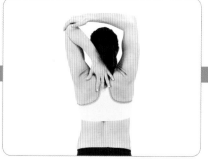

❾ Triceps Stretch, page 114

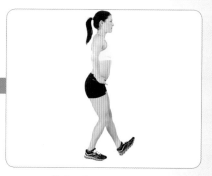

❿ Calf Stretch, page 116

POSTURAL PICK-ME-UP

This routine works your primary and secondary chest muscles as well as your core and lower back. As much as possible, keep your spine in neutral, neither arched nor hunched forward; when bending over as in Dead Lift, move smoothly and with control.

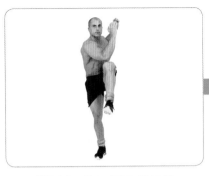

1 Twisting Knee Raise, page 48

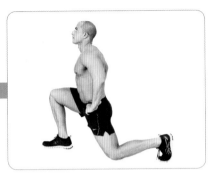

2 Jumping Lunge, page 36

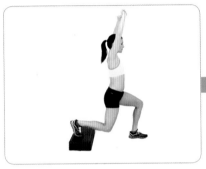

3 Split Squat with Overhead Press, page 30

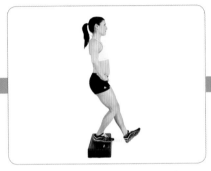

4 One-Legged Step-Down, page 42

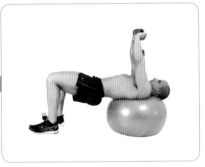

5 Swiss Ball Pullover, page 88

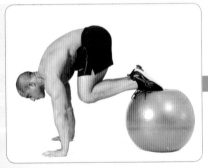

6 Swiss Ball Jackknife, page 38

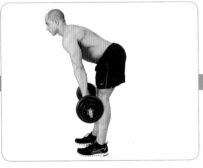

7 Dead Lift, page 80

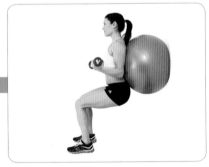

8 Ball Squat with Biceps Curl, page 90

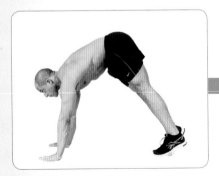

9 Arm-Reach Plank, page 46

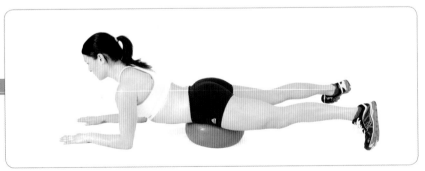

10 Heel Beat, page 50

STRENGTHEN & LENGTHEN

Activated arms and legs plus a pulled-in belly will help you carry out this full-body workout. Keep movements controlled, focus on balance, and stop if you find yourself jerking, slumping, or hunching.

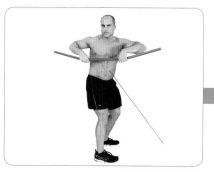

❶ Twisting Lift, page 102

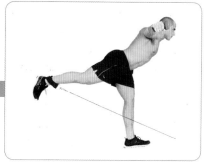

❷ Hip Extension with Reverse Fly, page 110

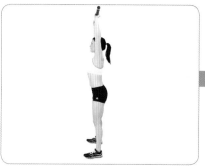

❸ Clean and Press, page 66

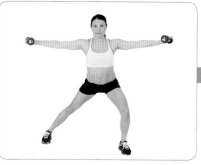

❹ Lateral-Extension Lateral Lunge, page 72

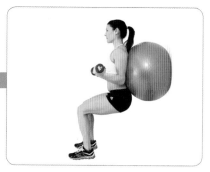

❺ Ball Squat with Biceps Curl, page 90

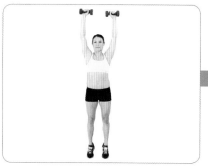

❻ Toe Raise with Overhead Press, page 70

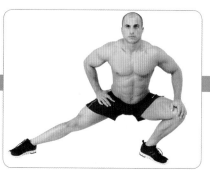

❼ Side Adductor Stretch, page 128

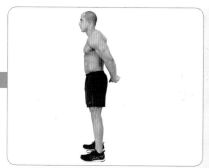

❽ Pectoral Stretch, page 115

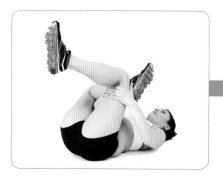

❾ Piriformis Stretch, page 118

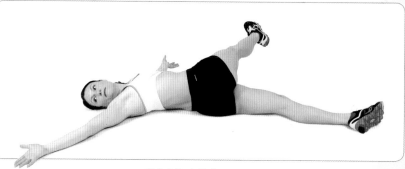

❿ Full-Body Roll, page 60

BACK CARE SEQUENCE

Your back supports the majority of your functional activities, whether you are swinging a tennis racket or sitting in a driver's seat. Treat it well with these movements, and remember: if an activity causes strain, back off.

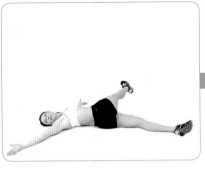

❶ Full-Body Roll, page 60

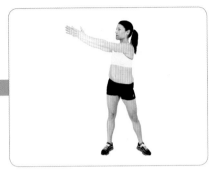

❷ Diagonal Reach, page 22

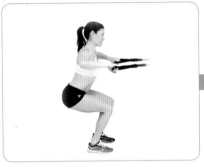

❸ Squat and Row, page 104

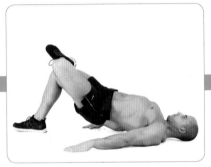

❹ Piriformis Bridge, page 54

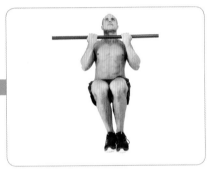

❺ Chin-Up with Hanging Leg Raise, page 58

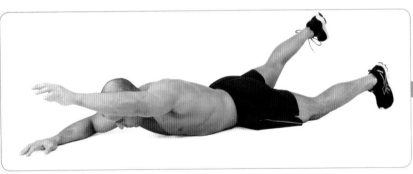

❻ Swimming, page 52

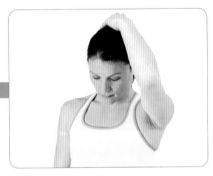

❼ Neck Flexion, page 123

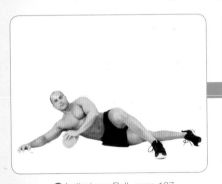

❽ Latissimus Roll, page 137

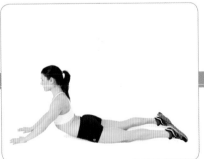

❾ Cobra Stretch, page 130

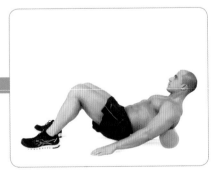

❿ Back Roll, page 140

TENSION BUSTER

When you sense stress or stiffness in your body, turn to this stretching, releasing workout for relief.

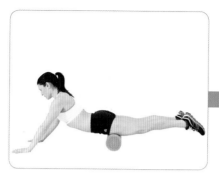

❶ Quadriceps Roll, page 134

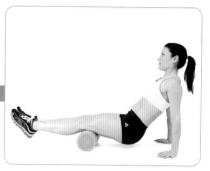

❷ Hamstrings Roll, page 135

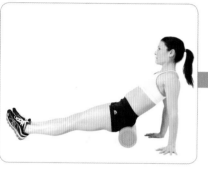

❸ Gluteal Roll, page 136

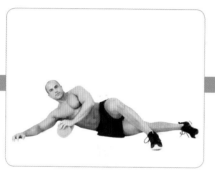

❹ Latissimus Roll, page 137

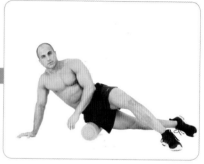

❺ Tensor Fasciae Latae Roll, page 138

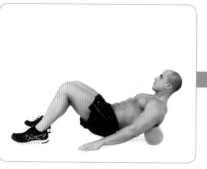

❻ Back Roll, page 140

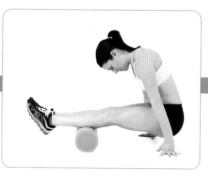

❼ Thread the Needle, page 142

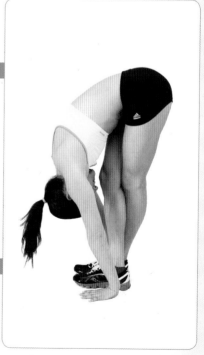

❽ Neck Flexion, page 122

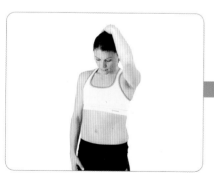

❾ Neck Side Bend, page 123

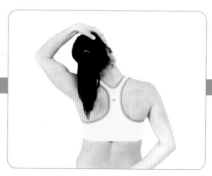

❿ Iliotibial Band Stretch, page 124

153

WEIGHT-ROOM ROUNDUP

Approach the weight room the Functional Training way: if you find your form suffering, switch to a different exercise rather than adding more and more repetitions.

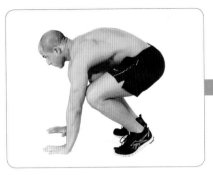

1 Functional Burpee, page 32

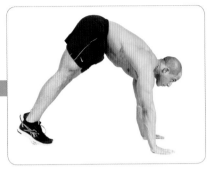

2 Push-up Walkout, page 44

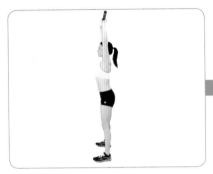

3 Clean and Press, page 66

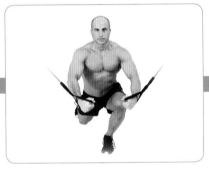

4 Reverse Lunge with Chest Press, page 106

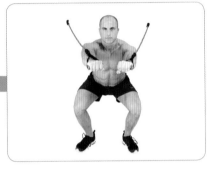

5 Press and Squat, page 108

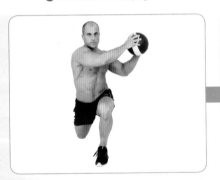

6 Reach-and-Twist Walking Lunge, page 64

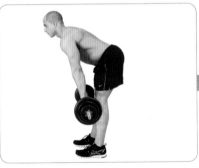

7 Dead Lift, page 80

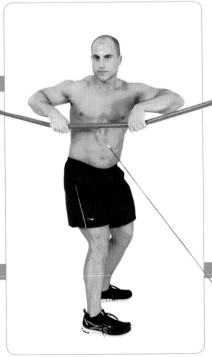

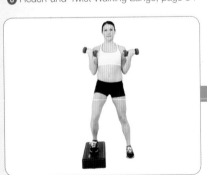

8 Lateral Step and Curl, page 92

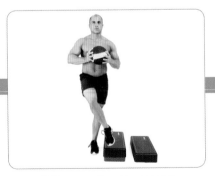

9 Crossover Step-Up, page 94

10 Twisting Lift, page 102

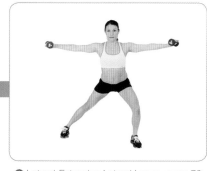

11 Lateral-Extension Lateral Lunge, page 72

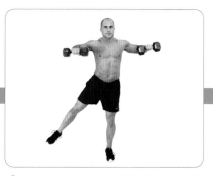

12 Knee Raise with Lateral Extension, page 78

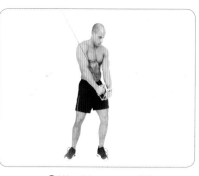

13 Woodchop, page 100

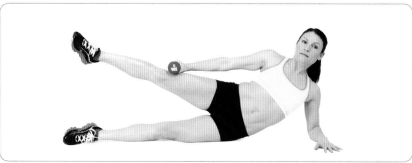

14 Lying Abduction, page 84

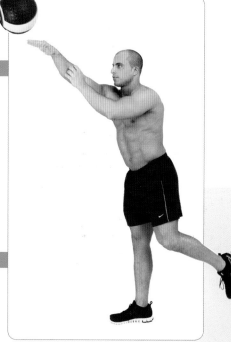

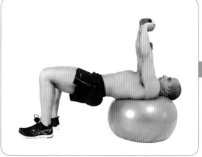

15 Swiss Ball Pullover, page 88

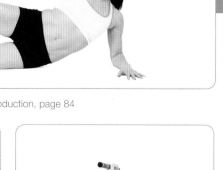

16 Roll-up Triceps Lift, page 82

17 Knee-Flexion Ball Throw, page 68

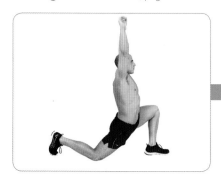

18 Hip-to-Thigh Stretch, page 120

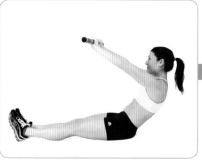

19 Triceps Stretch, page 114

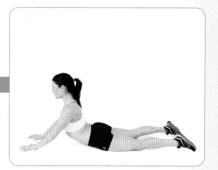

20 Cobra Stretch, page 130

BODY BALANCER

Practised in sequence, this workout will cultivate your sense of balance. Keep breathing, inhaling to prepare and exhaling as you execute the moves. Picture yourself growing leaner, stronger, and more centered as you work.

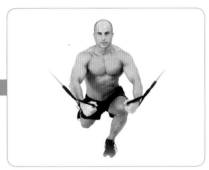

1 Twisting Knee Raise, page 48

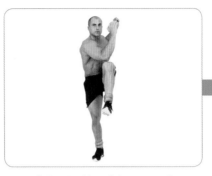

2 Reverse Lunge with Chest Press, page 106

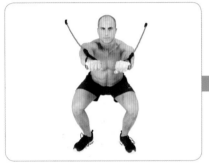

3 Press and Squat, page 108

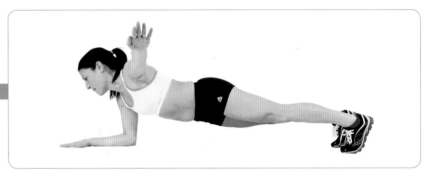

4 Arm-Reach Plank, page 46

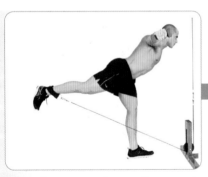

5 Hip Extension with Reverse Fly, page 110

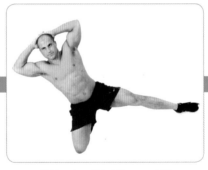

6 Kneeling Side Lift, page 132

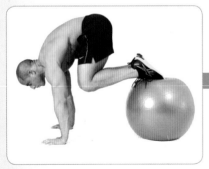

7 Swiss Ball Jackknife, page 38

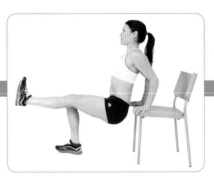

8 Leg-Extension Chair Dip, page 40

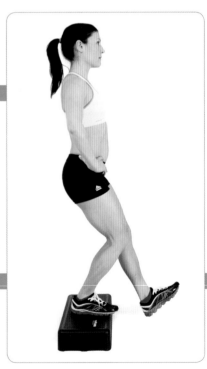

9 One-Legged Step-Down, page 42

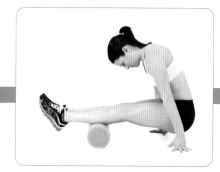
⑩ Thread the Needle, page 142

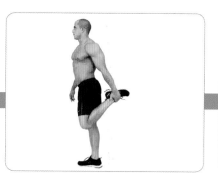
⑪ Quadriceps Stretch, page 117

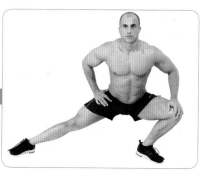
⑫ Side Adductor Stretch, page 128

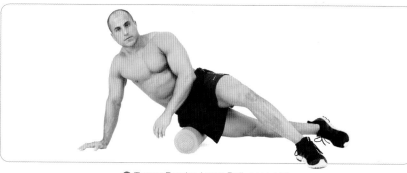
⑬ Tensor Fasciae Latae Roll, page 138

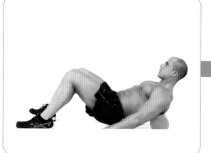
⑭ Back Roll, page 140

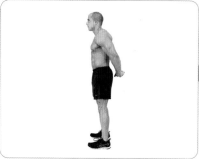
⑮ Pectoral Stretch, page 115

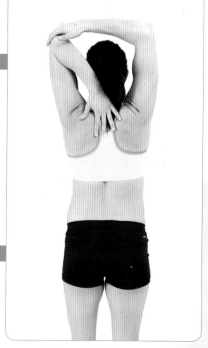
⑯ Triceps Stretch, page 114

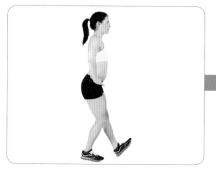
⑰ Calf Stretch, page 116

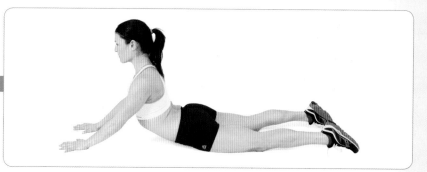
⑱ Cobra Stretch, page 130

GLOSSARY

GENERAL TERMS

abduction: Movement away from the body.

adduction: Movement towards the body.

anterior: Located in the front.

cardiovascular exercise: Any exercise that increases the heart rate, making oxygen and nutrient-rich blood available to working muscles.

cardiovascular system: The circulatory system that distributes blood throughout the body; it includes the heart, lungs, arteries, veins and capillaries.

core: Refers to the deep muscle layers that lie close to the spine and provide structural support for the entire body. The core is divisible into major core and minor core. The major-core muscles are on the trunk and include the belly area and the mid- and lower back. This area encompasses the pelvic-floor muscles (levator ani, pubococcygeus, iliococcygeus, pubo-rectalis and coccygeus), the abdominals (rectus abdominis, transversus abdominis*, obliquus externus and obliquus internus*), the spinal extensors (multifidus spinae*, erector spinae*, splenius*, longissimus thoracis and semispinalis*) and the diaphragm. The minor core muscles include the latissimus dorsi, gluteus maximus and trapezius (upper, middle and lower). These minor core muscles assist the major muscles when the body engages in activities or movements that require added stability.

crunch: A common abdominal exercise that calls for curling the shoulders towards the pelvis while lying supine with your hands behind the head and your knees bent.

curl: An exercise movement, usually targeting the biceps brachii, that calls for a weight to be moved through an arc, in a 'curling' motion.

dead lift: An exercise movement that calls for lifting a weight, such as a barbell, off the ground from a stabilised bent-over position.

dumbbell: A basic piece of equipment that consists of a short bar on which weight plates are secured. A person can use a dumbbell in one or both hands during an exercise. Most gyms offer dumbbells with the weight plates welded on and the number of kilograms indicated on the plates, but many dumbbells intended for home use come with removable plates that allow you to adjust the weight.

dynamic exercise: An exercise that includes movement through the joints and muscles.

extension: The act of straightening.

extensor muscle: A muscle serving to extend a body part away from the body.

flexion: The bending of a joint.

flexor muscle: A muscle that decreases the angle between two bones, such as bending the arm at the elbow or raising the thigh towards the stomach.

fly: An exercise movement in which the hand and arm move through an arc while the elbow is kept at a constant angle. A fly works the muscles of the upper body.

iliotibial band (ITB): A thick band of fibrous tissue that runs down the outside of the leg, beginning at the hip and extending to the outer side of the tibia, just below the knee joint. The ITB works in conjunction with several of the thigh muscles to provide stability to the outside of the knee joint.

lateral: Located on, or extending towards, the outside.

medial: Located on, or extending towards, the middle.

medicine ball: A small weighted ball that is used in weight training and toning.

neutral position (spine): A spinal position resembling an S shape, consisting of a lordosis (backward curvature) in the lower back, when viewed in profile.

posterior: Located behind.

press: An exercise movement that calls for moving a weight, or other resistance, away from the body.

range of motion: The distance and direction a joint can move between the flexed position and the extended position.

resistance band: Any rubber tubing or flat band device used for strength training that provides a resistive force. Also called a 'fitness band', 'stretching band' and 'stretch tube'.

rotator muscle: One of a group of muscles that assist the rotation of a joint, such as the hip or the shoulder.

scapula: The protrusion of bone on the mid- to upper back. Also known as the 'shoulder blade'.

squat: An exercise that calls for moving the hips back and bending the knees and hips to lower the torso (and an accompanying weight, if desired) and then returning to the upright position. A squat primarily targets the muscles of the thighs, hips and buttocks, as well as the hamstrings.

static exercise: An isometric form of exercise, without movement of the joints, where a position is held for a specific period of time.

Swiss ball: A flexible, inflatable PVC ball, measuring approximately 35 to 86 centimetres in circumference, used for weight training, physical therapy, balance training and other exercise regimens. It is also called a 'balance ball', 'fitness ball', 'stability ball', 'exercise ball', 'gym ball', 'physioball', 'body ball' and many other names.

warm-up: Any form of light exercise of short duration that prepares the body for more intense activity.

weight: Refers to the plates or weight stacks, or the actual poundage listed on the bar or dumbbell.

LATIN TERMS

The following glossary explains the Latin terminology used to describe the body's musculature. Where words are derived from the Greek, this is indicated.

CHEST

coracobrachialis*: Greek korakoeidés, 'ravenlike', and brachium, 'arm'

pectoralis (major and minor):

pectus, 'breast'

ABDOMEN
obliquus externus: obliquus, 'slanting', and externus, 'outwards'

obliquus internus*: obliquus, 'slanting', and internus, 'within'

rectus abdominis: rego, 'straight, upright', and abdomen, 'belly'

serratus anterior: serra, 'saw', and ante, 'before'

transversus abdominis*: transversus, 'athwart, across', and abdomen, 'belly'

NECK
scalenus*: Greek skalénós, 'unequal'

semispinalis*: semi, 'half', and spinae, 'spine'

splenius*: Greek splénion, 'plaster, patch'

sternocleidomastoideus: Greek stérnon, 'chest', Greek kleís, 'key', and Greek mastoeidés, 'breastlike'

BACK
erector spinae*: erectus, 'straight', and spinae, 'spine'

latissimus dorsi: latus, 'wide', and dorsum, 'back'

multifidus spinae*: multifid, 'to cut into divisions', and spinae, 'spine'

quadratus lumborum*: quadratus, 'square, rectangular', and lumbus, 'loin'

rhomboideus*: Greek rhembesthai, 'to spin'

trapezius: Greek trapezion, 'small table'

SHOULDERS
deltoideus anterior: Greek deltoeidés, 'delta-shaped' (that is, triangular), and ante, 'before'

deltoideus medialis: Greek deltoeidés, 'delta-shaped' (that is, triangular), and medialis, 'middle'

deltoideus posterior: Greek deltoeidés, 'delta-shaped' (that is, triangular), and posterus, 'behind'

infraspinatus*: infra, 'under', and spinae, 'spine'

levator scapulae*: levare, 'to raise', and scapulae, 'shoulder [blades]'

subscapularis*: sub, 'below', and scapulae, 'shoulder [blades]'

supraspinatus*: supra, 'above', and spinae, 'spine'

teres (major and minor): teres, 'rounded'

UPPER ARM
biceps brachii: biceps, 'two-headed', and brachium, 'arm'

brachialis: brachium, 'arm'

triceps brachii: triceps, 'three-headed', and brachium, 'arm'

LOWER ARM
anconeus: Greek anconad, 'elbow'

brachioradialis: brachium, 'arm', and radius, 'spoke'

extensor carpi radialis: extendere, 'to extend', Greek karpós, 'wrist', and radius, 'spoke'

extensor digitorum: extendere, 'to extend', and digitus, 'finger, toe'

flexor carpi pollicis longus: flectere, 'to bend', Greek karpós, 'wrist', pollicis, 'thumb', and longus, 'long'

flexor carpi radialis: flectere, 'to bend', Greek karpós, 'wrist', and radius, 'spoke'

flexor carpi ulnaris: flectere, 'to bend', Greek karpós, 'wrist', and ulnaris, 'forearm'

flexor digitorum*: flectere, 'to bend', and digitus, 'finger, toe'

palmaris longus: palmaris, 'palm', and longus, 'long'

pronator teres: pronate, 'to rotate', and teres, 'rounded'

HIPS
gemellus (inferior and superior): geminus, 'twin'

gluteus maximus: Greek gloutós, 'rump', and maximus, 'largest'

gluteus medius*: Greek gloutós, 'rump', and medialis, 'middle'

gluteus minimus*: Greek gloutós, 'rump', and minimus, 'smallest'

iliacus*: ilium, 'groin'

iliopsoas*: ilium, 'groin', and Greek psoa, 'groin muscle'

obturator externus: obturare, 'to block', and externus, 'outwards'

obturator internus*: obturare, 'to block', and internus, 'within'

pectineus*: pectin, 'comb'

piriformis*: pirum, 'pear', and forma, 'shape'

quadratus femoris*: quadratus, 'square, rectangular', and femur, 'thigh'

UPPER LEG
adductor longus: adducere, 'to contract', and longus, 'long'

adductor magnus: adducere, 'to contract', and magnus, 'major'

biceps femoris: biceps, 'two-headed', and femur, 'thigh'

gracilis*: gracilis*, 'slim, slender'

rectus femoris: rego, 'straight, upright', and femur, 'thigh'

sartorius: sarcio, 'to patch, to repair'

semimembranosus: semi, 'half', and membrum, 'limb'

semitendinosus: semi, 'half', and tendo, 'tendon'

tensor fasciae latae: tendere, 'to stretch', fasciae, 'band', and latae, 'laid down'

vastus intermedius*: vastus, 'immense, huge', and intermedius, 'between'

vastus lateralis: vastus, 'immense, huge', and lateralis, 'side'

vastus medialis: vastus, 'immense, huge', and medialis, 'middle'

LOWER LEG
adductor digiti minimi: adducere, 'to contract', digitus, 'finger, toe', and minimum 'smallest'

adductor hallucis: adducere, 'to contract', and hallex, 'big toe'

extensor digitorum: extendere, 'to extend', and digitus, 'finger, toe'

extensor hallucis: extendere, 'to extend', and hallex, 'big toe'

flexor digitorum*: flectere, 'to bend', and digitus, 'finger, toe'

flexor hallucis*: flectere, 'to bend', and hallex, 'big toe'

gastrocnemius: Greek gastroknémía, 'calf [of the leg]'

peroneus: peronei, 'of the fibula'

plantaris: planta, 'sole'

soleus: solea, 'sandal'

tibialis anterior: tibia, 'reed pipe', and ante, 'before'

tibialis posterior*: tibia, 'reed pipe', and posterus, 'behind'

trochlea tali: trochleae, 'pulley-shaped structure', and talus, 'lower portion of ankle joint'

PHOTOGRAPHY
Photography by FineArtsPhotoGroup.com
Models: Joseph Benedict, Jillian Langenau

ILLUSTRATIONS
All large illustrations by Hector Aiza/3D Labz Animation India, except the insets throughout and the full-body anatomy art works on pages 12 and 13: by Linda Bucklin/Shutterstock.

ACKNOWLEDGEMENTS
The author and publisher also offer thanks to those closely involved in the creation of this book: Moseley Road President Sean Moore, General Manager Karen Prince, art director Tina Vaughan and production director Adam Moore; and designer Heather McCarry.

ABOUT THE AUTHORS

Erica Gordon-Mallin

Growing up, Erica Gordon-Mallin would have chosen the library over the gym any day. But now, as a writer and seasoned fitness book editor, she is delighted to have found functional training, with its focus on how we move our whole bodies in real life. She finds the results wonderfully effective, and intends to follow this fitness approach for many years to come. A graduate of Amherst College and University College London, Erica lives in Manhattan.

Erica's Acknowledgements

A big thank you to Lisa Purcell, whose work in developing this series laid the groundwork for Anatomy of Functional Training and so many other books still to come. Big thanks also to Hollis Liebman who advised on the muscle diagrams, coming through with flying colours on short notice. Thank you to Danielle Scaramuzzo for her early design work. And on a personal note, I would like to thank my always-supportive father, Sam Mallin; my grammar inspiration, Marion Wolfthal; and Mariel Gold, my sister and best friend.

Katerina Spilio

At the age of 16, Katerina Spilio began climbing on scaffolding to decorate church ceilings with her father. The need for strength, flexibility and endurance became quickly apparent and led to a lifelong fitness career. As a personal trainer certified by the Aerobics and Fitness Association of America, over 30 years she has taught countless group classes and individual sessions---most recently at Rye Personal Fitness and Mind and Body Fitness in New York. A firm believer in the mind-body connection, she continues to motivate and train people in functional exercise, while also maintaining her ecclesiastic artwork studio in Dobbs Ferry, New York.

Katerina's Acknowledgements

I would like to thank my father, the late Reverend John Spilio who taught me to exercise every day of my life, and my mother Mary, ever svelte and fit, who provides an incredible role model. Thanks also to my daughters Ariadne and Alexandra for whom I always strive to be a better person.